THE 90-DAY

weight
training
plan

THE 90-DAY
weight training plan

AN EFFECTIVE WORKOUT AND NUTRITION PROGRAM TO BUILD MUSCLE AND MAXIMIZE ENERGY

JULIE GERMAINE CORAM

ILLUSTRATION BY CHANTEL DE SOUSA

ROCKRIDGE
PRESS

Interior and Cover Designer: Peatra Jariya
Art Producer: Tom Hood
Editor: Andrea Leptinsky
Production Editor: Rachel Taenzler

Illustration © Chantel de Sousa, 2020

ISBN: Print 978-1-64739-816-3 | eBook 978-1-64739-491-2
R0

TO MY SWEETEST BABY GIRL, AMELIA.
FOREVER MY FAVORITE WORKOUT PARTNER!

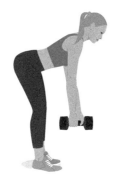

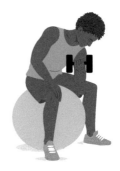

contents

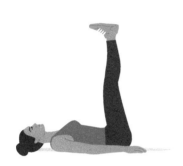

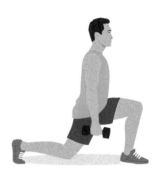

Introduction

Welcome!

I am Julie Germaine Coram, a mother and a health coach with nearly two decades' experience helping thousands of people get into the best shape of their lives.

My passion for fitness led me to compete for 12 years, graduating from an amateur athlete to a professional fitness model. I won multiple international Pro shows, was runner-up at the World Beauty Fitness and Fashion Championships, and landed magazine covers and countless fitness instruction spreads.

My career also allowed me to shine the spotlight on my amazing client transformations and inspire others to push their personal limits and believe that they, too, could build their dream body.

Since giving birth to my daughter, Mia, in 2018, I have a whole new respect for the female body. I loved pregnancy and embraced all the changes I experienced, but I had to work hard to regain my former shape and learn how to balance motherhood and my active lifestyle. Switching it up to exercise at home was a game changer for me—and I am happy to share my most effective workouts with you!

By reading this book, you will develop a better understanding of how the body works to build muscle, and how to eat for your fitness goals. The book makes nutrition simple, with easy to understand week-by-week guides that show you carb timing, appropriate protein intake, and food choices to build lean muscle mass.

You can achieve amazing results exercising in your own home if you know how to properly challenge your body during weight training. This book will show you how to set up your home gym and will teach you the best moves to create a balanced, symmetrical physique. Better yet, you'll also get tips on how to keep your progress going and push past training plateaus.

How to Use This Book

This book shows you how to build a fantastic physique. Part 1 covers important fundamentals of weight training that will help you understand the process. This foundation will motivate you to work harder and earn those gains! Goal setting, tracking results, choosing the right equipment, and training safely are all necessary topics to review before beginning any fitness program.

The meat of the book is in part 2. This is the training and nutrition plan—a detailed and targeted program that makes getting into sculpted shape a sure thing. Here you will find three months of workouts, complete with training fundamentals and tips on achieving the intensity and skill you need to promote change in your body. To help you eat well, the nutrition plan is broken down according to your protein requirements and activity level, with helpful grocery lists and meal suggestions.

Finally, part 3 allows you to have Coach Julie right there with you! This is a reference section that covers all the weight exercises listed in part 2, to ensure your form is correct and you are training your body effectively.

Why 90 Days?

You may wonder why I chose the 90-day format. I've used this timeline throughout my entire career as a personal trainer. One reason is because it takes time to embrace a new lifestyle and see results from a training regimen. First, you have to go through a preparation phase to ready the body for intense exercise. This preparation phase reconditions the body, increases lean muscle mass, and boosts short-term endurance. As you move into a bulking phase to allow your body to grow stronger, you need time to adjust to more challenging workouts. Luckily, you'll be encouraged by fast results as the weeks progress—a newbie to weight training could put a few inches on their arms within 90 days!

Yes, You Can

This program can work for you. Yes, YOU! The workouts are customizable for all athletes, from beginner to advanced. I'll help you easily understand the movements, guiding you on exercise technique, proper form, and training intensity to get amazing results. While your current goal might be to change your appearance by building muscle and getting leaner, you will also make positive improvements to your general health at the same time.

Disclaimer

All the material in this book is presented with the intent of giving helpful information on weight training, fitness, nutrition, and related topics. This book should not be used to diagnose or treat any medical condition. You should always speak with your doctor before beginning a fitness program or making a change to your activity level, especially if you answer yes to any of the following:

- You have a heart condition.

- You feel pain in your chest, whether or not you are doing a physical activity.

- You lose your balance because of dizziness or loss of consciousness.

- You have a joint or bone problem that could be made worse by a change in your physical activity.

- You are on doctor-prescribed drugs for high blood pressure or a heart condition.

- You are pregnant.

For diagnosis or treatment of any medical problem, please consult your physician. Rockridge Press and the author are not responsible for any specific health or allergy needs that may require medical supervision and warn you to closely consider the dietary recommendations before making personal adjustments. Individuals with eating disorders or other food-related medical conditions should consult with a doctor before making a change to their diets. Those involved in this project are not liable for damages or any negative consequences from any action, treatment, application, or preparation to any person reading or following the information in the book. References provided are for informational purposes only and don't constitute endorsement of any websites or other sources. Readers should understand that websites listed in this book could possibly change.

PART I

BEFORE YOU START

Whether or not you have weight training experience, the information in this section is essential. Fully understanding the basics of weightlifting will drastically improve your results and reduce your risk of injury. I take my job as your coach seriously, and want to help you get started on a safe and healthy path.

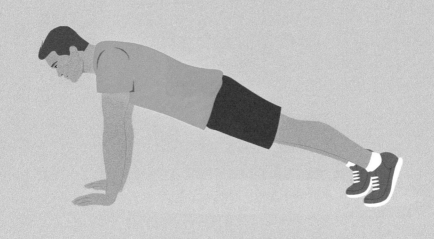
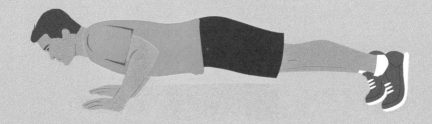

The Basics

1

In this chapter, you'll learn how your body responds to, and recovers from, weight training. This knowledge will help you make sense of the techniques in subsequent chapters and will guide you in establishing realistic fitness goals.

The Science of Weight Training

Exercise does wonders for your body, but—I'll be honest—it's going to feel really tough at the beginning, and it should. Why? Because weight training actually damages your muscles. During each challenging rep, microscopic tears develop in the muscle belly. A newbie to lifting will be particularly sore two days after the workout, which is called DOMS, or delayed onset muscle soreness. This pain indicates the body's response to the trauma—it repairs the muscle tissue to become stronger than it was before.

Rest days play an important role in exercise, whether you're trying to lose weight or build muscle, because rest encourages your muscles to rebuild and grow. It's also a good idea to follow a structured workout program that works specific muscle groups together. Your training split should provide tired body parts with regular breaks, as well as a few full days off from training.

Once your muscles recover, it's time to do it all again. As the body adapts to the new activity, your job is to continue to nudge your capabilities along by pushing yourself harder than you did in your last workout, then patiently allow the muscles to relax and expand. This process will ensure you are consistently seeing improvements in your physical appearance and athletic performance.

Setting Personal Goals

Goal setting is key to success, so spend time journaling about what your motivation to weight train is, what your goals are, and how you expect to get there. Envision how you'll feel after 12 successful weeks of dedicated training and healthy eating. Close your eyes and let yourself experience that pride and sense of accomplishment—visualization will help you make your dreams a reality. You can use this technique to motivate yourself whenever you need it.

Creating realistic goals that take into consideration the bodybuilding process is extremely valuable. Strength gains can be impressive in the beginning stages of a fitness program—as much as 20 to 30 percent. In terms of muscle development, that would equal about one to two pounds of lean muscle mass. If your goal is to increase in size, it will be a little more difficult to calculate within our 90-day timeline. It's tough to say how long it will take to put an inch on your biceps until you chart your personal results, but you can definitely expect to build them. Keep in mind that while you're putting on muscle, you're also becoming leaner or losing body fat. Muscle and fat tissues take up space differently in the body, so remember this when assessing your weight and measurements to help you establish new and attainable fitness goals.

Tracking Your Progress

Progress photos—along with measurements, body fat percentages (if possible), and strength improvements—are a useful way to gauge fitness results. Tracking your progress from day one takes less than five minutes. It also helps you evaluate your efforts and success as the weeks pass and encourages you to keep going. Photos should be taken of you standing relaxed in swimwear, in the same place, and at the same time of day to ensure consistency in room lighting and physique. Mornings are usually the best. When you wake up, before you eat breakfast, take measurements while flexed (e.g., bend your arm to flex your biceps, or press downward to flex your quadriceps in your legs). Stand tall but relaxed when taking your core measurement—shoulders back, breathe in and then out slowly, measuring right over your belly button without sucking in or letting your belly hang out. You can refer to the chart at the end of the book (see page 183) to guide you further on how to complete your assessment. For useful week-by-week strength charts, please visit my website for the free download (see the Resources on page 185).

Getting the Right Equipment

Setting up a home gym should be fun. Depending on your fitness level, it's possible to put on quality muscle without investing too much money. Many calisthenics exercises will help you build a strong base, but having some essential equipment for weightlifting will ensure you keep making progress.

To begin building your home gym, I recommend purchasing the following:

- A mat
- Tension bands (or glute bands) for the thighs/hips, in varying resistance levels (see my preferred set at juliegermaine.com)
- Weight training gloves (to help you securely grip the weights and save your hands from blisters)
- A stability ball
- Three sets of dumbbells, ranging from 5 to 20 pounds

This is the minimum equipment you'll need to follow the weight training program in the coming chapters. As your strength improves and you are able to lift heavier loads, you should graduate to a stable workout bench to safely push bigger weights. Other optional accessories you can purchase to add intensity to your workout include a BOSU ball or balance board, medicine balls, a pull-up bar, and if you live in a climate that endures a harsh winter, a piece of cardio equipment.

See the Resources section for a source for finding this required equipment, as well as direct links to posts on other topics at juliegermaine.com.

Staying Safe

There is potential for serious injury with resistance training if done incorrectly. Learning proper form is extremely important for beginners, but advanced athletes can also benefit from a review of their technique. Be sure to keep safety at the top of your mind throughout this program.

Part 3 provides expert instruction for each movement to help you develop a strong and safe foundation. It also covers variations for each fitness level to help you find what's right for you. If you completely understand which body part is being used and how the exercise should feel, you'll get rewards from each movement.

At the same time, resist falling into a fitness routine that feels too comfortable. Keep pushing your body to change by increasing the intensity of your workouts. A good sign that your workouts are not challenging enough is when you stop experiencing DOMS as much.

Here's another guideline for exercise intensity: If I were there with you to spot your bench press, and let's say you were on your eighth rep, would you be able to do four more without my help or encouragement to keep going? If the answer is yes, that's an indication that you need to increase the amount of weight you are lifting.

As you start lifting heavier weights in your workouts with the progressive overload principle, you'll find that your technique will actually change somewhat. Your body will first become familiar with the range of motion, allowing you to push your muscles closer to failure. "Failure," in this case, is a bodybuilding term that's actually positive. It refers to fatiguing your muscle belly during exercise to the point where it cannot continue to lift even one more repetition. Training "to failure" is not always appropriate, but getting close to this outcome is important because it cues the body to strengthen the area.

Before you begin any lift, allow your full mental focus to be on the exercise and pay attention to a strong core setup. Next, be aware of your body positioning and of maintaining muscle contraction during the lift. Your tempo will vary depending on the exercise, whether you have a spotter to assist you, and your goal with the workout.

Above all, train safely—you're never quite the same after an injury, so be patient, learn as you go, and never rush into a new exercise without knowing the correct technique.

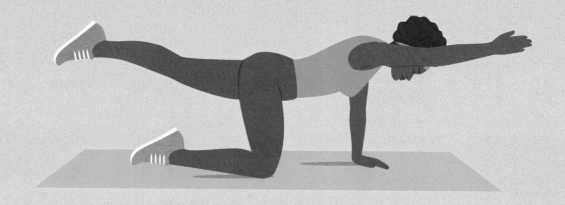

ESSENTIAL TECHNIQUES

2

To optimize your training performance and maximize your muscle building results, pay close attention to each element of your workout. Breathing correctly will improve your strength and endurance by circulating oxygenated blood. Setting your body up properly before each set will protect your spine and increase your overall success by effectively targeting the correct muscle groups during the movement. Following the guideline for repetitions and sets for each training cycle will appropriately fatigue the muscle belly to prepare it for growth. Using the right amount of weight and adhering to the progressive overload principle for individual exercises will keep you from hitting training plateaus and ensure you consistently make progress.

Breathing

Controlling your breathing during each repetition can take time to master, but the effort is worth it. New trainees often hold their breath when working through a challenging set, but this can be dangerous because it decreases blood flow to the heart. This drop in blood pressure can lead to sudden unconsciousness from the reduced blood supply to the brain. You could also experience dizziness, become disoriented, and do potential damage when gasping for air again. Individuals with a heart condition are particularly vulnerable to spikes in blood pressure, and retinal hemorrhages can occur when the blood vessels behind the eyes are strained. The best practice is to breathe in during the eccentric portion of the exercise (when you're lowering the weight with gravity), and exhale during the concentric movement (when you're exerting yourself physically to lift).

Proper Form

If you want to enjoy the long-term benefits of an active lifestyle, you need to learn the proper form for every exercise. Not only will this protect you against sudden or repetitive-use injury, but training correctly will amplify your results and encourage you to keep going! Knowing how to position and move your body is easier when you have an understanding of the muscles you are targeting. You'll learn about this in the step-by-step instructions for each exercise in part 3. Here are some general lifting techniques to get you started:

- One of the most important factors to always keep in mind is protecting your spine:
  - › Never arch your back.
  - › Engage your abdominals before beginning the lift.
  - › Keep your neck in a comfortable neutral position.
- Your posture should be strong, with shoulders set back and chest open.
- Balance your feet firmly (supportive, appropriate footwear is important, even when training in your home).
- During lower-body exercises, such as squats:
  - › Sit back into the exercise, pushing your butt out as if you were lowering into a chair.

> Your knees shouldn't extend past your toes, because that position puts additional strain on your joints.

> Distribute your weight through your heels rather than on the balls of your feet.

Reps/Sets

In weight training, we talk in terms of reps (repetitions), sets, rest, and tempo. A repetition refers to one complete movement through a particular exercise. This takes you from the starting position, through the full range of both concentric and eccentric motion, and back to the beginning.

A set is the number of reps you group together before resting. The length of a set depends on your fitness goal. In this book, sets for muscle building will typically be in the 8 to 12 rep range. When developing strength during peak week (the timeframe in which you reach your optimal physical condition), this will reduce to 1 to 3 reps. Athletes focused on endurance, on the other hand, would push themselves to repeat the exercise 30 to 60 times, sometimes even more. The muscle should be working under stress throughout the entire set and should only relax during the rest period. Rests between sets are a chance to catch your breath and give the targeted muscles a moment to recover before you challenge them again.

Tempo is the length of time it takes to move your body during each exercise. Slowing down can make the workout more difficult, and explosive, fast movements can make the body adapt in response. Tempo in muscle building programs is often outlined as 3:1:1, or 3 seconds eccentric, 1 second isometric (no movement occurring), and 1 second concentric.

Proper Weight Amounts

To develop maximum strength and increase your muscle mass, you need to push your body. Think of yourself as a beautiful, efficient machine. The goal when bodybuilding is to fatigue the muscle belly so your body knows it needs to be stronger in that area. You have to (safely) push yourself near failure; otherwise, the body will see no need to adapt.

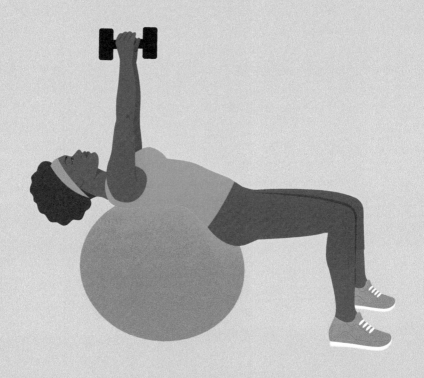

The importance of nutrition

3

Getting in shape and staying fit require you to develop good habits to support your health objectives. The types of foods and the amounts you consume have a direct impact on how you will look and feel. Weight training adds more activity to your day, which burns more calories during and after the workout. Providing your body with the nutrients it needs to properly repair muscle tissue and grow means paying close attention to when and what you eat. If your diet is lacking, your results will be, too.

Essential Nutritional Guidelines

Fortunately, you don't need to drive yourself crazy obsessing over calories or figuring out your macronutrient ratio for every meal as you start your weight training plan. The nutrition plan in the chapters ahead makes eating well straightforward and manageable.

Protein is the building block of muscle. It's made up of amino acids that are responsible for growing, repairing, and maintaining your body's tissues. Complete proteins—which come from foods such as red meat, poultry, fish, eggs, and dairy—are easiest for your body to digest. But you may also find it convenient to use whey, soy, or casein protein powders to boost your daily intake of protein.

Carbohydrates (carbs) are essential in a bulking diet and help repair muscles. You'll find these sugars, starches, and fibers in fruits, grains, milk products, and vegetables. Sugar promotes an increase in insulin levels, which helps transport nutrients into the muscle cells. Fruit contains two types of sugar: fructose and glucose, which can easily be converted into fat. Consuming fresh fruit instead of starches leads to a lower insulin response. This is beneficial for maintaining a healthy, lean physique, decreasing the risk of disease and increasing your overall quality of life.

Fats are essential to everyone's diet—including athletes. They help with vitamin absorption, promote brain health, protect your organs, help keep you warm, and give your body energy to support cell growth. Adding healthy fats to your diet will make you feel satisfied for longer, reducing hunger. There is also a benefit to eating a higher protein and fat meal before a workout. This can shift your metabolism from burning glucose to burning stored fat for energy during exercise, which will make developing a fit body more achievable. Food absorption slows when fat is introduced, so there's more time to use food for energy during training and before the body stores these calories as fat.

Avocados, olives, nuts, peanut butter, soybeans, and tofu all contain healthy fats. Limit foods that are high in saturated fats, like beef, chicken with skin, and some cheeses.

Here are some great options for a healthy, nutritious pre-workout meal:

- Omega-3-enriched eggs (poached, hard-boiled, or scrambled) with spinach and onion

- Rice cakes with cream cheese and smoked salmon

- Baked or grilled salmon with sweet potatoes and grilled vegetables

- Pita and hummus

- Avocado toast with chicken slices

- Cottage cheese with nut butter and crushed walnuts

Snack options include:

- Beef jerky

- Rice crackers with natural peanut butter

- Protein shake and almonds

- Protein bar

It's crucial to a muscle building program to have a steady source of protein throughout the day, but it's particularly important to infuse protein immediately post-workout, ideally within 20 minutes of completing your final rep. Pairing this protein with a fast-acting carb will kick-start muscle development. Here are some perfect meals to consume after your strength training:

- Grilled chicken with sweet potatoes and vegetables

- Tuna wrap with lettuce and tomato

- Nonfat cottage cheese bowl with sliced fruit

- Oatmeal with whey protein and banana

- Turkey, potatoes, and steamed vegetables

- Whole wheat pasta with chicken and tomato sauce

Snack options include:

- A glass of chocolate milk and an apple

- Greek yogurt with fruit

- Tuna and crackers

The body is about 60 percent water. To prevent dehydration, you need to drink adequate amounts of water. Sip on water constantly throughout the day, even when you're not thirsty, to keep your energy level up and your brain functioning in high gear.

SUPPLEMENTS

Supplements are a great way to improve your fitness results! Of course, the best way to get the vitamins and nutrients your body needs to build muscle is via food—there are no pills to fix a bad diet. But supplements, such as protein powder, glutamine, BCAAs (branched-chain amino acids), creatine, and multivitamins, can help improve your muscle recovery and amplify your workouts. It's best to start with one supplement at a time and watch for any adverse effects before adding another one.

PART II

THE NUTRITION AND TRAINING PLAN

You're now ready to get to work building your dream body! The next four chapters provide you with a complete nutrition and weight training program with the primary objective of gaining muscle. To achieve fantastic results, you will need to practice good nutrition and weight training together. Your body needs the proper nutrients to build muscle, and you need the right foods to fuel epic workouts. After just a few days of following the diet plan, you will feel more energetic and have fewer sugar cravings. Many of my clients also experience better sleep and less stress within their first weeks of exercise.

ASSESSMENTS

At this point, I highly recommend recording your weight and taking measurements using the information provided on page 5. Throughout this part of the book, you will be prompted to do assessments to guide you in making dietary decisions that support and encourage your training efforts. Small improvements add up as the weeks go by, but you have to take notes to be sure your body is changing. You can also visit juliegermaine.com/90-day -plan to download a free chart that lets you track your overall strength gains before each assessment.

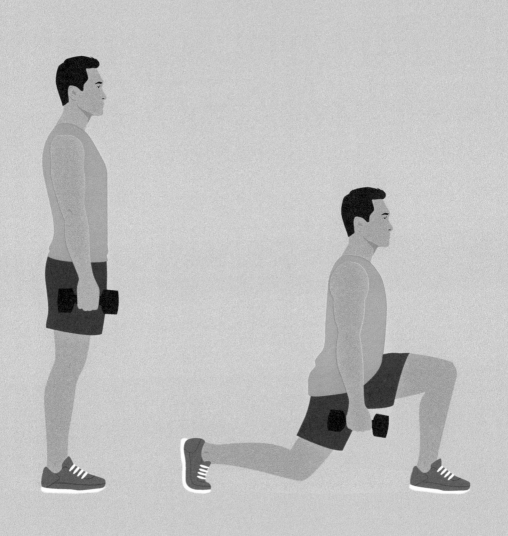

weeks 1 to 3: general preparation

4

This chapter guides your body through a general preparation that eases you into more intense training. Introducing your body to this program gradually is important to allow your metabolism to improve and to give your muscles time to adjust to the increased activity level. Each movement will feel more natural week by week as you take the time to learn proper form and do higher repetitions to establish muscle memory, build short-term endurance, and increase overall strength. To develop lean muscle mass during this phase, you will want to complete 3 to 5 sets using a light weight and aim for 8 to 15 repetitions per set.

Nutrition Plan

This week is dedicated to eating the right amount of calories to build muscle based on your body type. To gauge the appropriate serving size for protein and carbs, use your hand as a guide. Meat protein, such as a steak or chicken breast, should be about the size and thickness of your palm. Carbohydrates, like sweet potatoes or brown rice, should fit into your cupped hand. Vegetables and leafy greens can be enjoyed without limitation, and you are encouraged to snack on them throughout the day.

SHOPPING LIST FOR THE WEEK

- For meat: choose from canned light tuna, skinless chicken breast, lean steak, turkey bacon, bison, salmon
- For vegetarians: choose from tofu, soy milk, tempeh
- Coconut oil spray
- Dark chocolate
- Foods containing healthy fats: avocados, pistachios, natural peanut butter, peanuts, edamame beans, chia seeds
- Fiber One cereal
- Fruit: apples, berries, bananas, raisins
- Hummus
- Light cream cheese
- Low-glycemic carbohydrates: sweet potatoes, oats, pumpernickel bread, potatoes, whole-wheat pasta
- Nonfat salad dressings
- Omega-3-enriched eggs and a carton of egg whites
- Protein powder, low-carb variety
- Salsa
- Skim milk

- Spices

- Sugar-free Jell-O

- Tomato sauce

- Whole-wheat bagels

- Whole-wheat pitas

- Vegetables: cauliflower, carrots, sun-dried tomatoes, bell peppers, asparagus, romaine lettuce

- Vegetable soup

MEAL PLAN FOR THE WEEK

Breakfast Options

- 3 whole omega-3-enriched eggs and 2 egg whites, avocado, berries, Fiber One cereal with skim milk

- 6 slices turkey bacon, oatmeal with double serving of natural peanut butter, and ¼ cup raisins

- 2 whole omega-3-enriched eggs and 2 egg whites with salsa, 2 slices turkey bacon or tempeh, whole-wheat bagel with light cream cheese

Lunch Options

- Light tuna salad pita pocket

- Chicken, side of vegetables, slice of pumpernickel bread or potatoes

- Tofu, vegetable soup with chia seeds, sweet potatoes

Dinner Options

- Large serving of steak or bison with vegetables, sweet potatoes or potatoes, and a square of dark chocolate

- Salmon over whole-wheat pasta with tomato sauce and greens, sugar-free Jell-O

- Edamame beans, veggies with hummus, pistachios, dark chocolate

HOW DO I CALCULATE MY ESTIMATED CALORIC INTAKE?

Visit juliegermaine.com /90-day-plan to find out what your estimated caloric intake should be to build muscle. You will find a helpful calculator you can use. Doing this will help you personalize this shopping list to your needs and will set you up for fantastic results. You can also browse the many healthy recipes there to get great ideas for your own meals.

Post-Workout Options

- 1 to 2 scoops protein powder mixed in water and a banana

- Protein powder mixed in skim milk and berries

- Protein powder blended with soy milk and half a frozen banana

DAILY CALORIE, PROTEIN, AND CARB RECOMMENDATIONS

As a guideline, the average basal metabolic rate (BMR), also known as basal energy expenditure (BEE), for women is around 1,400 calories, while for men it's about 1,800. You must take into consideration your increased activity level due to workouts, plus add extra calories if you want to gain muscle. This would bring your recommended caloric intake closer to 2,200 to 2,400 for women and 2,600 to 2,800 for men. For maximum strength gains, 1 gram of protein per pound of body weight is best, or 2.2 grams of protein per kilogram of body weight.

Day-by-Day Routines

Focus Lower Body

Muscles quadriceps, glutes, hamstrings, calves, core muscles (rectus abdominis, internal and external obliques, transverse abdominals, erectors)

Length of Workout 10 to 15 minutes

Repetitions 3 sets each exercise, 12 to 15 reps

Beginner Workout squats (warm-up sets), squats (working sets), lunges, glute hip thrusts, calf raises, wall sits (cool-down)

Intermediate Workout add 3 working sets of squats with bands (sets available at juliegermaine.com)

Advanced Workout add leg curls

> **Warm-ups** are essential before weight training; they reduce the risk of tears or strains by preparing the joints for activity.

Week 1, Day 2

Rest Day

> **Fit TIP**
> I recommend sweating every day! Active recovery on rest days can mean going for a brisk walk or a bike ride to get the blood and the endorphins flowing.

Week 1, Day 3

Focus Upper Body

Muscles pectorals, deltoids, triceps, latissimus dorsi, rhomboids, biceps, core muscles (rectus abdominis, internal and external obliques, transverse abdominals, erectors)

Length of Workout 10 to 15 minutes

Repetitions 3 sets each exercise, 12 to 15 reps

Beginner Workout push-ups (warm-up), shoulder presses, single-arm dumbbell rows, bicep curls, dips (cool-down)

Intermediate Workout add pulldowns

Advanced Workout add overhead tricep extensions

> ### Fit TIP
> Stay hydrated and energized by sipping water as you rest after each set.

Week 1, Day 4

Rest Day

Week 1, Day 5

Focus Core

Muscles rectus abdominis, internal and external obliques, transverse abdominals, erectors, hip flexors

Length of Workout 10 to 15 minutes

Repetitions 3 sets each exercise, 12 to 15 reps

Beginner Workout bird dogs (warm-up), band bicycle crunches, leg raises, butterfly crunches, planks with shoulder tap (cool-down)

Intermediate Workout add V-sit twists

Advanced Workout add side planks with torso twist

> ### Food TIP
> Your post-workout meal should be consumed within 20 minutes of completing your last set.

Week 1, Day 6

Repeat Day 1 or Rest Day

Week 1, Day 7

Rest Day

Nutrition Plan

Making the transition to eating whole, unprocessed foods can be a struggle for many people, so don't be discouraged if your diet was not 100 percent healthy last week. This week, the goal is to continue to embrace your healthy lifestyle and promote muscle growth by trying new foods to broaden your palate and discover the best meal plan for you.

SHOPPING LIST FOR THE WEEK

- For meat: choose from lean steak, turkey, bison, tilapia or other white fish, salmon
- For vegetarians: choose from seitan, almond milk, lentils, pinto beans
- Foods containing healthy fats: walnuts, hemp hearts
- Fruit: cantaloupe, grapes, grapefruit, peaches
- Light cheddar cheese
- Light granola bars (like Nature Valley)
- Light popcorn
- Low-glycemic carbohydrates: sweet potatoes, wild rice, pumpernickel bread
- Nonfat Greek yogurt
- Omega-3-enriched eggs
- Protein powder, low-carb
- Vegetables: broccoli, green and yellow squash, green beans, tomatoes, cucumbers, snap peas, romaine lettuce, potatoes

MEAL PLAN FOR THE WEEK

Breakfast Options

- Yogurt with walnuts, grapes, granola bar

- 2 whole scrambled eggs with light cheddar, pumpernickel toast, grapefruit

- Glass of almond milk, grapes, walnuts, and a granola bar

Lunch Options

- Turkey with a mixed green salad and wild rice

- Tilapia with mixed vegetables and pumpernickel bread

- Lentils or pinto beans with vegetables and Greek yogurt

Dinner Options

- Large serving of steak or bison with vegetables, sweet potatoes

- Salmon with salad, wild rice

- Seitan (optional), mixed greens with hemp hearts, and sweet potatoes or wild rice

Post-Workout Options

- 1 to 2 scoops protein powder mixed in water and a piece of fruit

Evening Snack

- Popcorn

DAILY CALORIE, PROTEIN, AND CARB RECOMMENDATIONS

You will want to maintain a consistent caloric intake for a number of weeks and assess your results before drastically changing your diet. When your primary goal is muscle development, a macronutrient ratio of 40 to 60 percent carbohydrates, 25 to 40 percent protein, and 15 to 20 percent fats is optimum.

Day-by-Day Routines

Focus Upper Body

Muscles pectorals, deltoids, triceps, latissimus dorsi, rhomboids, biceps, core muscles (rectus abdominis, internal and external obliques, transverse abdominals, erectors)

Length of Workout 10 to 15 minutes

Repetitions 3 sets each exercise, 12 to 15 reps

Beginner Workout Supermans (warm-up), shoulder presses, pulldowns, overhead tricep extensions, plank walks (cool-down)

Intermediate Workout add glute kickbacks

Advanced Workout add calf raises

> **Safety Advice**
> With any overhead weight training exercise, it's a good idea to use a spotter. If you are exercising alone, be sure to lift only what you can control and have a phone within reach, as unforeseen accidents can happen and you may need to call for help.

Week 2, Day 2

Rest Day

Week 2, Day 3

Focus Lower Body

Muscles quadriceps, glutes, hamstrings, calves, core muscles (rectus abdominis, internal and external obliques, transverse abdominals, erectors)

Length of Workout 10 to 15 minutes

Repetitions 3 sets each exercise, 12 to 15 reps

Beginner Workout squats (warm-up), deadlifts, leg curls, leg abductions, wall sits (cool-down)

Intermediate Workout add double-grasp rows

Advanced Workout add concentration curls

> ### Fit TIP
> Rest periods between sets should be just long enough to catch your breath—less than a minute.

Week 2, Day 4

Rest Day

Week 2, Day 5

Focus Core

Muscles rectus abdominis, internal and external obliques, transverse abdominals, erectors

Length of Workout 10 to 15 minutes

Repetitions 3 sets each exercise, 12 to 15 reps

Beginner Workout bird dogs (warm-up), V-sit twists, leg raises, push presses, planks with shoulder tap (cool-down)

Intermediate Workout add Supermans

Advanced Workout add butterfly crunches

> ### Food TIP
> Space your meals out every three to four hours to boost your metabolism and reduce body fat. Your metabolism speeds up after you eat, so graze on nutrient-rich snacks between big meals.

Week 2, Day 6

Repeat Day 1 or Rest Day

Week 2, Day 7

Rest Day

Nutrition Plan

To make strength gains, be sure to adjust your caloric intake to account for improvements to your metabolism. By consuming regular nutritious meals throughout the day and doing a regular exercise routine, your body burns more calories. This week, your overall food intake has been slightly increased to encourage consistent progress.

SHOPPING LIST FOR THE WEEK

- For meat: choose from canned light tuna, lean sirloin steak, pork tenderloin, turkey, halibut, smoked salmon
- For vegetarians: choose from tofu, soybeans, seitan
- Foods containing healthy fats: almonds, pumpkin seeds, natural peanut butter
- Fruit: dried fruit, apples, watermelon, berries
- Gluten-free crackers
- Light cream cheese
- Low-glycemic carbohydrates: brown rice, quinoa, oats, whole-wheat pasta, whole-wheat bread, whole-wheat wraps
- Natural fruit jam, no sugar added
- Nonfat cottage cheese
- Omega-3-enriched eggs
- Protein bars, low-fat/low-carb
- Protein powder, low-carb
- Sugar-free pudding
- Vegetables: cauliflower, celery, fennel, tomatoes, bell peppers, spinach, romaine lettuce

MEAL PLAN FOR THE WEEK

Breakfast Options

- Large serving of top sirloin with 2 omega-3-enriched eggs, oatmeal, and dried fruit

- Seitan, 2 eggs (optional), 1 to 2 servings whole-wheat bread with 2 tablespoons jam

Snack Options

- Apple and 1 to 2 tablespoons natural peanut butter

- 1 cup cottage cheese, ½ cup berries, and handful of almonds or pumpkin seeds

Lunch Options

- Canned light tuna or turkey with salad and pasta with tomatoes

- Tofu vegetable wrap

Snack Options

- Protein bar

- 8 crackers with 6 ounces smoked salmon and 2 tablespoons light cream cheese

Dinner Options

- Medium serving of pork tenderloin, tossed salad with brown rice, and sugar-free pudding

- Halibut or soybeans with mixed vegetables, large serving of quinoa, and sugar-free pudding

Post-Workout Option

- 1 to 2 scoops protein powder mixed in water and a piece of fruit

DAILY CALORIE, PROTEIN, AND CARB RECOMMENDATIONS

Total calories for each day are about 200 higher, spread out over more meals. This week, the macronutrient percentages are not dramatically different, but your carbohydrate intake has been increased slightly to provide your body the fuel necessary for the important task of muscle regeneration.

Day-by-Day Routines

Focus Lower Body

Muscles quadriceps, glutes, hamstrings, calves, core muscles (rectus abdominis, internal and external obliques, transverse abdominals, erectors)

Length of Workout 10 to 15 minutes

Repetitions 3 sets each exercise, 12 to 15 reps

Beginner Workout squats (warm-up), squats (working sets), glute kickbacks, calf raises, wall sits (cool-down)

Intermediate Workout add glute hip thrusts

Advanced Workout add leg curls

> **Safety Advice**
> As you try to increase strength, gradually push yourself to use heavier weights, but never sacrifice proper form.

Week 3, Day 2

Rest Day

Week 3, Day 3

Focus Push and Core

Muscles pectorals, deltoids, triceps, internal and external obliques, transverse abdominals, erectors

Length of Workout 10 to 15 minutes

Repetitions 3 sets each exercise, 12 to 15 reps

Beginner Workout push-ups (warm-up), shoulder presses, bird dogs, bent-arm lateral raises, dips (cool-down)

Intermediate Workout add butterfly crunches

Advanced Workout add chest flys

> ## Fit TIP
> You have an assessment coming up! Always be sure to record your lifts (number of reps and size of weights) during your workouts the week before your assessment so you can make note of your strength improvements when you review your physical results. Visit juliegermaine.com/90-day-plan for free charts.

Week 3, Day 4

Rest Day

Week 3, Day 5

Focus Pull and Core

Muscles latissimus dorsi, rhomboids, biceps, abdominals, internal and external obliques, transverse abdominals, erectors

Length of Workout 10 to 15 minutes

Repetitions 3 sets each exercise, 12 to 15 reps

Beginner Workout Supermans (warm-up), single-arm rows, side planks with torso twist, pullovers, standing reverse flys (cool-down)

Intermediate Workout add straight-arm pushdowns

Advanced Workout add pull-ups

> ## Food TIP
> Taking a multivitamin every day can ensure your body is topped up with essential vitamins and minerals for better health and a stronger body. Also, food prep makes eating healthy so much easier! If you haven't already embraced this routine, give it a try and marvel at how much more time you have in the day when your meals are packaged and ready to eat in just a few minutes.

Week 3, Day 6

Repeat Day 1 or Rest Day

Week 3, Day 7

Rest Day

Time for a Weigh-In

The moment of truth has arrived! Please go to page 183 and complete your first reassessment. It will be interesting to compare your current weight, measurements, and photos to those you collected before you began the nutrition and training program. Understanding the subtle ways your body has changed will motivate you to keep going, and help you decide if you need to adjust your caloric intake to improve future results. For help assessing your results, or if you'd like to share your progress with someone, please reach out to me online! I love hearing from my clients, and I'm here to serve as a resource throughout your fitness journey.

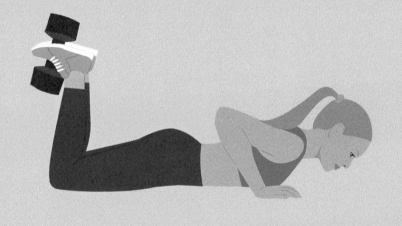

weeks 4 to 6: Building Basic strength

5

Over the past three weeks, you have developed muscle memory that will give you a fantastic foundation for your strength training. This means you're ready to move forward and challenge your body with heavier sets to establish power and increase muscle size. These workouts will take you through specific strength movements that will prepare you for future high-intensity work. Warm-ups and cool-downs should always be done at high repetitions (15 or more). During this phase, you will best improve your muscle density by performing 3 to 5 working sets using moderate to heavy weights and completing 8 to 12 repetitions.

Nutrition Plan

It is always a good idea to revisit your nutrition plan after an assessment and make adjustments based on your results. Each body is unique and should be treated as such. If you enjoyed great results and are feeling stronger and looking leaner and fuller, then wonderful job! Your diet plan will continue to work for you over the following weeks. If you unexpectedly lost weight, increase your overall calories by adding to your servings of carbs and protein in two of your meals, or by enjoying a high-protein snack before bed. If you feel you have gained some body fat, reduce your carbohydrate intake in one or two meals later in the day. Increasing cardiovascular exercise will also help fat melt away.

SHOPPING LIST FOR THE WEEK

- For meat: choose from shrimp, skinless chicken breast, lean steak, bison

- For vegetarians: tempeh, almond milk

- Foods containing healthy fats: avocados, natural peanut butter, peanuts, edamame beans

- Fruit: olives, bananas, grapes, kiwi

- Light cheddar, mozzarella, or goat cheese

- Low-glycemic carbohydrates: quinoa, wild rice, pumpernickel bread, whole-wheat pasta, potatoes

- Mini-Wheats cereal

- Nonfat Greek yogurt

- Protein powder, low-carb

- Skim milk

- Vegetables: spinach, broccoli, celery, fennel, green beans, bell peppers, asparagus

MEAL PLAN FOR THE WEEK

Breakfast Options

- 1 to 2 scoops protein powder blended with 1 cup skim milk and kiwi, and Home-made Protein Pancakes (recipe, including a list of the ingredients you'll need, is available at juliegermaine.com/fitness-blog)

- Mini-Wheats cereal with almond milk, fruit, and 2 scoops protein powder mixed in water

Snack Options

- Avocado pumpernickel toast (recipe available at juliegermaine.com/fitness-blog)

- Edamame beans

Lunch Options

- Roasted shrimp or chicken and vegetable skewers with potatoes

- Quinoa salad bowl with goat cheese

Dinner Options

- Bison or lean steak with double serving of vegetables and wild rice

- Tempeh and whole-wheat vegetable pasta

Snack Options

- Protein ice cream (1 scoop protein powder, 1 tablespoon natural peanut butter)

- Nonfat Greek yogurt and peanuts

Post-Workout Option

- 1 to 2 scoops protein powder mixed in water and a piece of fruit

DAILY CALORIE, PROTEIN, AND CARB RECOMMENDATIONS

Eating smaller meals throughout the day helps raise your metabolism and keeps hunger at bay. You should customize the meals to your food preferences and adjust the servings to align with your goals and assessment results.

Day-by-Day Routines

Week 4, Day 1

Focus Quadriceps and Glutes

Muscles quadriceps, glutes, core muscles (rectus abdominis, internal and external obliques, transverse abdominals, erectors)

Length of Workout 10 to 15 minutes

Repetitions 3 sets each exercise, 8 to 12 reps

Beginner Workout squats (warm-up), lunges, glute kickbacks, glute hip thrusts, wall sits (cool-down)

Intermediate Workout add 3 additional working sets of squats

Advanced Workout add leg abductions

> ### Safety Advice
> Bingeing is bad for your health, so limit your indulgences to moderate amounts of food, stop the cheating after one meal, and return immediately to your healthy food plan. Check out restaurant menus online ahead of time if you are going out to eat so you can make your healthy choice before you're too hungry.

Week 4, Day 2

Focus Chest, Shoulders, Triceps, and Abdominals

Muscles pectorals, deltoids, triceps, rectus abdominis, transverse abdominals

Length of Workout 10 to 15 minutes

Repetitions 3 sets each exercise, 8 to 12 reps

Beginner Workout bent-arm lateral raises (warm-up), Arnold presses, chest flys, dips, plank walks (cool-down)

Intermediate Workout add chest presses

Advanced Workout add push presses

Fit TIP

The shoulder joint should be protected by moving only within a natural range of motion. Never overextend or rotate your arm under stress. Performing exercises with a tempo of 3:1:1, or 3 seconds eccentric (lowering with gravity), 1 second isometric (no movement occurring), 1 second concentric (lifting against gravity), can make the workout more difficult.

WHAT IS A DROP-SET?

A drop-set is when you immediately pick up a lighter (but still challenging) weight and perform additional sets to fail, then rest, and repeat the entire process again. Also called burnout sets, this style of training is exceptionally effective for strength improvement, especially when you add even more drop-sets to push yourself, reducing the weight three or four times.

Week 4, Day 3

Rest Day

Week 4, Day 4

Focus Hamstrings and Calves

Muscles hamstrings, quadriceps, glutes, calves, core muscles (rectus abdominis, internal and external obliques, transverse abdominals, erectors)

Length of Workout 10 to 15 minutes

Repetitions 3 sets each exercise, 8 to 12 reps

Beginner Workout squats (warm-up), deadlifts, leg curls, calf raises, wall sits (cool-down)

Intermediate Workout add side-lying hip raises

Advanced Workout add drop-sets to all sets of deadlifts

Food TIP

Your body needs some fats from food, so be sure to eat "good" fats every day, such as avocado, olives, peanut butter, or walnuts. Trans fats clog your arteries, increase bad cholesterol, and reduce good cholesterol, so cut out the cookies, crackers, French fries, processed foods, and creamers.

Week 4, Day 5

Rest Day

Week 4, Day 6

Focus Back, Biceps, Obliques

Muscles latissimus dorsi, rhomboids, trapezius, biceps, internal and external obliques

Length of Workout 10 to 15 minutes

Repetitions 3 sets each exercise, 8 to 12 reps

Beginner Workout Supermans (warm-up), double-grasp rows, pull-ups or pulldowns, band bicycle crunches, standing reverse flys (cool-down)

Intermediate Workout add bicep curls

Advanced Workout add V-sit twists

> ### Safety Advice
> Getting outside to exercise is fun, but be weather-aware and dress to keep your body nice and toasty. Cold muscles are more susceptible to tears.

Week 4, Day 7

Rest Day

Nutrition Plan

Now that you have been strictly following your meal plan for a full month, you deserve to reward yourself with an off-diet treat meal. Food is one of the joys of life, so including your favorites once in a while is important. You can incorporate cheat meals every week or two to help you combat cravings and kick-start your metabolism, and doing so is encouraged as you continue your healthy, active lifestyle. This week's nutrition plan recommends calories be reduced somewhat to allow for this indulgence.

SHOPPING LIST FOR THE WEEK

- For meat: choose from skinless chicken breast, turkey bacon, lean ham
- For vegetarians: choose from tofu, tempeh, black beans, soy milk
- Dark chocolate
- Foods containing healthy fats: avocados, almonds, walnuts, chia seeds
- Fruit: pineapple, raspberries, kiwi, peaches
- Light cheddar cheese
- Light cream cheese
- Low-glycemic carbohydrates: sweet potatoes, pumpernickel bread, whole-wheat pasta, potatoes
- Nonfat Greek yogurt
- Omega-3-enriched eggs and carton of egg whites
- Protein powder, low-carb
- Rice cakes
- Vegetables: broccoli, green and yellow squash, carrots, celery, cucumbers, tomatoes, bell peppers, snap peas, romaine lettuce
- Vegetable soup

MEAL PLAN FOR THE WEEK

Breakfast Options

- 3 whole eggs and 2 egg whites, pineapple slices, and sweet potato hash browns
- 2-slice grilled cheese sandwich with 4 of the slices turkey bacon

Snack Options

- Plain nonfat Greek yogurt with celery and half an avocado
- Rice cakes with light cream cheese and cucumber

Lunch Options

- Chicken with vegetables and potatoes
- Tempeh with vegetable soup and chia seeds

Snack Options

- 1 square dark chocolate and almonds
- Kiwi and walnuts

Dinner Options

- Lean ham with roasted green and yellow squash and sweet potatoes
- Tofu or black beans mixed with assorted vegetables over pasta

Post-Workout Options

- 1 to 2 scoops protein powder mixed in water and a piece of fruit
- 1 to 2 scoops protein powder mixed in unsweetened soy milk

DAILY CALORIE, PROTEIN, AND CARB RECOMMENDATIONS

The total calories per day is reduced by only about 100 if the lunchtime carb serving is cut in half. This allows over 700 calories per week to be saved for your cheat meal, so you can enjoy it without worrying about gaining body fat. Or you could eat a full serving for lunch and reduce your carbohydrates at dinner. It's best to consume most of your calories around the time of your workout, so base your decision on when you typically exercise.

Day-by-Day Routines

Week 5, Day 1

Focus Quadriceps, Glutes

Muscles quadriceps, glutes, core muscles (rectus abdominis, internal and external obliques, transverse abdominals, erectors)

Length of Workout 10 to 15 minutes

Repetitions 3 sets each exercise, 8 to 12 reps

Beginner Workout squats (warm-up), squats (working sets), leg abductions, glute hip thrusts, wall sits (cool-down)

Intermediate Workout add lunges

Advanced Workout add glute kickbacks

> ### Fit TIP
> Stay consistent! Have a routine so you continue to hit the gym regularly. By now, you will start to see measurable improvements in your strength and fitness, so keep charting your lifts in your workout journal (available for free download at juliegermaine.com/90-day-plan) and make small increases week by week.

Week 5, Day 2

Rest Day

Week 5, Day 3

Focus Chest, Shoulders, Triceps, Core

Muscles pectorals, deltoids, triceps, rectus abdominis, transverse abdominals

Length of Workout 10 to 15 minutes

Repetitions 3 sets each exercise, 8 to 12 reps

Beginner Workout bird dogs (warm-up), chest presses, incline presses, overhead tricep extensions, planks with shoulder tap (cool-down)

Intermediate Workout add bent-arm lateral raises

Advanced Workout add leg raises, try planks using BOSU ball or push-ups with feet on a balance board

> ## Food TIP
> Saturated fats, like beef, chicken with skin, and cheese, should be limited to 5 percent of your daily calories.

Week 5, Day 4

Focus Hamstrings, Calves

Muscles hamstrings, glutes, quadriceps, calves, core muscles (rectus abdominis, internal and external obliques, transverse abdominals, erectors)

Length of Workout 10 to 15 minutes

Repetitions 3 sets each exercise, 8 to 12 reps

Beginner Workout squats (warm-up), deadlifts, leg curls, calf raises, wall sits (cool-down)

Intermediate Workout add drop-sets for all sets of leg curls or do 3 additional sets of leg curls

Advanced Workout add 3 additional sets of calf raises

> ## Safety Advice
> Maintaining a neutral spine is another valuable lesson that is applicable in every exercise. Planks strengthen your core and are a fantastic, full-body exercise! There are many ways to change it up to avoid getting bored and to keep your body guessing and adapting.

Week 5, Day 5

Rest Day

Week 5, Day 6

Focus Back, Biceps, Obliques

Muscles latissimus dorsi, rhomboids, trapezius, biceps, internal and external obliques

Length of Workout 10 to 15 minutes

Repetitions 3 sets each exercise, 8 to 12 reps

Beginner Workout Supermans (warm-up), pullovers, planks with torso twist, bicep curls, standing reverse flys (cool-down)

Intermediate Workout add concentration curls

Advanced Workout add double-grasp rows

> Fit TIP
>
> As you achieve goals, set yourself up with new benchmarks for your training to keep you motivated to work hard. Visualization will help you make your dreams a reality, so use this technique to motivate yourself often.

Week 5, Day 7

Rest Day

Nutrition Plan

You're doing such a great job and should be proud of yourself for successfully making it to Week 6! Keep your motivation soaring high and find new ways to make your healthy diet interesting by checking out some of the recipes available on my blog, juliegermaine .com/fitness-blog, and incorporating a variety of vegetables into your regimen.

SHOPPING LIST FOR THE WEEK*

- For meat: choose from skinless chicken breast, turkey, turkey bacon, lean ham, tilapia or other white fish
- For vegetarians: choose from tofu, tempeh, black beans, soy milk
- Dark chocolate
- Foods containing healthy fats: avocados, almonds, cashews, natural peanut butter, peanuts, walnuts, chia seeds
- Fruit: pineapple, raspberries, kiwi, peaches
- Hummus
- Light cheddar cheese
- Light cream cheese
- Low-glycemic carbohydrates: sweet potatoes, oats, pumpernickel bread, whole-wheat pasta, whole-wheat wrap, potatoes
- Nonfat cottage cheese
- Nonfat Greek yogurt
- Omega-3-enriched eggs and carton of egg whites
- Protein powder, low-carb
- Rice cakes

*The Week 6 shopping list is very similar to the list for Week 5. This similarity will aid you in getting more comfortable with maintaining a healthy diet.

- Skim milk
- Vegetables: broccoli, green and yellow squash, carrots, celery, cucumbers, tomatoes, bell peppers, snap peas, romaine lettuce
- Vegetable soup

MEAL PLAN FOR THE WEEK

This week you are doing almost the same meal plan as Week 5, with additional options for each meal.

Breakfast Options

- 3 whole eggs and 2 egg whites, pineapple slices, and sweet potato hash browns
- 2-slice grilled cheese sandwich with 4 of the slices turkey bacon
- 4 slices turkey bacon in a wrap with a kiwi and raspberries

Snack Options

- Plain nonfat Greek yogurt with celery and half an avocado
- Rice cakes with light cream cheese and cucumber
- Nonfat cottage cheese with 2 tablespoons peanut butter

Lunch Options

- Chicken with vegetables and potatoes
- Tempeh with vegetable soup and chia seeds
- Turkey with mixed greens salad and pumpernickel bread

Snack Options

- 1 square dark chocolate and almonds
- Kiwi and walnuts
- Peach and cashews

Dinner Options

- Lean ham with roasted green and yellow squash and sweet potatoes

- Tofu or black beans mixed with assorted vegetables over pasta

- Cashew-crusted tilapia served with fresh vegetable sticks dipped in hummus

Post-Workout Options

- 1 to 2 scoops protein powder mixed in water and a piece of fruit

- 1 to 2 scoops protein powder mixed in unsweetened soy milk

- 1 to 2 scoops protein powder blended with skim milk

DAILY CALORIE, PROTEIN, AND CARB RECOMMENDATIONS

Many of the muscle building meals you have been enjoying over the past five weeks can be staples in your diet after you complete this 12-week challenge! To continue to look and feel fantastic, make note of what nutritious foods you prefer, and develop your own healthy lifestyle.

Day-by-Day Routines

Focus Full Body

Muscles quadriceps, hamstrings, glutes, pectorals, latissimus dorsi, rhomboids, trapezius, deltoids, biceps, triceps, core muscles (rectus abdominis, internal and external obliques, transverse abdominals, erectors)

Length of Workout 10 to 15 minutes

Repetitions 3 sets each exercise, 8 to 12 reps

Beginner Workout push-ups (warm-up), squats (working sets), single-arm dumbbell rows, incline presses, dips (cool-down)

Intermediate Workout add shoulder press

Advanced Workout add pull-ups

> ## Food TIP
> Keep yourself from getting bored by changing up the protein, vegetables, and spices used with your diet plan. There are endless healthy recipes available online. Find even more recipes and fitness tips on my Instagram accounts: @sweatwithjulie and @julie.germaine or on facebook.com/sweatwithjulie.

Week 6, Day 2

Rest Day

Week 6, Day 3

Rest Day

Week 6, Day 4

Focus Chest, Back

Muscles pectorals, latissimus dorsi, rhomboids, trapezius, biceps, triceps, core muscles (rectus abdominis, internal and external obliques, transverse abdominals, erectors)

Length of Workout 10 to 15 minutes

Repetitions 3 sets each exercise, 8 to 12 reps

Beginner Workout Supermans (warm-up), double-grasp rows, chest presses, chest flys, standing reverse flys (cool-down)

Intermediate Workout add pullovers

Advanced Workout add push-ups

> ### Safety Advice
> Cooling down and doing a light stretch is great practice and will help your body recover more effectively. Supersets are perfect for effectively fatiguing your muscle bellies to encourage growth and compact your workout to make time for flexibility training. A superset is when you do one exercise and then immediately do a second one without resting, then rest and repeat both movements again.

Week 6, Day 5

Focus Legs

Muscles quadriceps, glutes, hamstrings, calves, core muscles (rectus abdominis, internal and external obliques, transverse abdominals, erectors)

Length of Workout 10 to 15 minutes

Repetitions 3 sets each exercise, 8 to 12 reps

Beginner Workout squats (warm-up), lunges, side-lying hip raises, glute hip thrusts, wall sits (cool-down)

Intermediate Workout add calf raises

Advanced Workout add leg abductions

> ### Fit TIP
> Fitness instructors often cue clients that their lunge form should result in both legs forming a 90-degree angle, but my experience has taught me that a straighter rear leg emphasizes the glutes during the movement and reduces knee strain on the back leg.

Focus Shoulders, Arms, Core

Muscles deltoids (anterior, medial, and posterior), pectorals, triceps, core muscles (rectus abdominis, internal and external obliques, transverse abdominals, erectors)

Length of Workout 10 to 15 minutes

Repetitions 3 sets each exercise, 8 to 12 reps

Beginner Workout bird dogs (warm-up), shoulder presses, bicep curls, planks with shoulder tap, dips (cool-down)

Intermediate Workout add lying one-arm lateral raises

Advanced Workout add overhead tricep extensions

> ## Food TIP
> Try to eat at home as much as possible so you are not tempted to eat high-calorie foods at a social get-together. Also, alcohol puts the brakes on fat burning while the liquid is metabolized by your body, so it's best to completely abstain while trying to achieve a new level of fitness.

Week 6, Day 7

Rest Day

> ## Time for a Weigh-In
> It's that time again! You've been working hard, so you should be eager to visit page 183 again to go through another fitness assessment. At times it may feel like nothing has changed, but that's why these check-ins are so critical. You'll prove to yourself that your efforts are well placed when you see the numbers moving in the right direction.

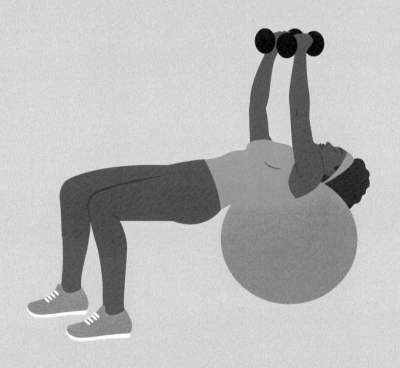

weeks 7 to 9: improving strength and power

6

The next three weeks are focused on continuing to build your muscle size and prepare you for greater power and strength. Your physical conditioning has improved immensely already, but these more difficult workouts and increasingly dialed-in nutrition plans will be challenging and may lead you to experience delayed onset muscle soreness. You should always try to perfect your lifting form and strive to increase the load used. During this phase, you will continue to improve your athleticism by doing 3 to 5 sets using moderate to heavy weights in the rep range of 8 to 12.

Nutrition Plan

Time to get real and start to cut out the foods that could be holding you back from achieving your full potential. To get lean while growing stronger, reduce the excess saturated fats, salt, and sugar that come from dairy. You will find that you can replace those fats with better options while keeping your calories at the same ideal muscle building level.

SHOPPING LIST FOR THE WEEK

- For meat: choose from canned light tuna, salmon, lean steak
- For vegetarians: choose from tofu, soybeans
- Foods containing healthy fats: avocados, edamame beans, hemp seeds, natural peanut butter
- Fruit: blueberries, limes, cantaloupe, honeydew melon
- Gluten-free crackers
- Low-glycemic carbohydrates: quinoa, oats, whole-wheat pasta
- Nonfat cottage cheese
- Omega-3-enriched eggs and carton of egg whites
- Protein bars, low-fat and low-carb
- Protein powder, low-carb
- Vegetable soup
- Vegetables: cauliflower, celery, green beans, cucumbers, sun-dried tomatoes, asparagus, butter lettuce
- Whole-wheat bread

MEAL PLAN FOR THE WEEK

Breakfast Options

- Protein powder mixed in water and toast with peanut butter

- 3 whole eggs and 2 egg whites and large serving of oatmeal with blueberries

Snack Options

- Protein bar

- Half an avocado with lime on crackers

Lunch Options

- Canned tuna with lettuce and fresh bread

- Tofu quinoa bowl with veggies

Snack Options

- Vegetable soup

- Edamame beans

Dinner Options

- Lean steak or salmon with asparagus and quinoa

- Soybeans, cauliflower, green beans, sun-dried tomatoes, and hemp seeds over pasta

Post-Workout Option

- 1 to 2 scoops protein powder mixed with water and a serving of fruit

DAILY CALORIE, PROTEIN, AND CARB RECOMMENDATIONS

If you're hungry for a pre-bed meal, please snack freely on crunchy vegetables like cauliflower, celery, or cucumbers, and enjoy another serving of lean protein, such as nonfat cottage cheese, chicken breast, or a protein shake made with water. You don't have to worry about deducting these calories from another meal.

Day-by-Day Routines

Focus Back, Glutes

Muscles latissimus dorsi, rhomboids, trapezius, biceps, glutes, quadriceps, core muscles (rectus abdominis, internal and external obliques, transverse abdominals, erectors)

Length of Workout 10 to 15 minutes

Repetitions 3 to 5 sets each exercise, 8 to 12 reps

Beginner Workout Supermans (warm-up), deadlifts, glute kickbacks, double-grasp rows, wall sits (cool-down)

Intermediate Workout add bird dogs

Advanced Workout add pulldowns

> ### Safety Advice
> Wearing gloves during weightlifting is particularly helpful on pull days, to keep your hands from developing painful blisters from the tug of the weights and to improve your grip on the handles. Putting on supportive shoes, even when training at home, helps you ground yourself during exercises and protect your feet. Reach out to me for where to find the best pair.

Focus Shoulders, Chest

Muscles deltoids, pectorals, triceps, core muscles (rectus abdominis, internal and external obliques, transverse abdominals, erectors)

Length of Workout 10 to 15 minutes

Repetitions 3 to 5 sets each exercise, 8 to 12 reps

Beginner Workout bent-arm lateral raises (warm-up), incline presses, chest flys, lying one-arm lateral raises, standing reverse flys (cool-down)

Intermediate Workout add plank walks

Advanced Workout add push-ups

> ### Fit TIP
> Guarantee a great workout by eating a meal about 30 to 60 minutes prior to weight training. To reap the benefit of cheat meals, eat them before a workout. You'll love the pumps to your muscles and the boost of energy you get from a carb-heavy dish.

Week 7, Day 3

Rest Day

Week 7, Day 4

Focus Arms, Core

Muscles pectorals, anterior deltoids, biceps, triceps, core muscles (rectus abdominis, internal and external obliques, transverse abdominals, erectors)

Length of Workout 10 to 15 minutes

Repetitions 3 to 5 sets each exercise, 8 to 12 reps

Beginner Workout push-ups (warm-up), bicep curls, push presses, overhead tricep extensions, dips (cool-down)

Intermediate Workout add concentration curls

Advanced Workout add bicycles

> ### Food TIP
> Feeling run-down? It might be time for a cheat meal to bomb your body with calories, boost your metabolism, and uplift your spirits!

Week 7, Day 5

Focus Quads, Hamstrings, Calves

Muscles quadriceps, glutes, calves, anterior deltoids, core muscles (rectus abdominis, internal and external obliques, transverse abdominals, erectors)

Length of Workout 10 to 15 minutes

Repetitions 3 to 5 sets each exercise, 8 to 12 reps

Beginner Workout squats (warm-up), lunges, leg curls, calf raises, plank walks (cool-down)

Intermediate Workout add 3 additional working sets of squats

Advanced Workout add 3 additional sets of leg curls

> ### Safety Advice
> Pace yourself as your body adjusts to these workouts. If the muscle group you are training is still sore from a previous workout, add an additional rest day so your body can fully recover.

Week 7, Day 6

Rest Day

Week 7, Day 7

Focus Back, Core

Muscles latissimus dorsi, rhomboids, trapezius, biceps, core muscles (rectus abdominis, internal and external obliques, transverse abdominals, erectors)

Length of Workout 10 to 15 minutes

Repetitions 3 to 5 sets each exercise, 8 to 12 reps

Beginner Workout Supermans (warm-up), straight-arm pushdowns, pull-ups or pullovers, single-arm dumbbell rows, planks with shoulder tap (cool-down)

Intermediate Workout add V-sit twists

Advanced Workout add leg raises

> ### Fit TIP
> Focus on learning how to properly engage your core before worrying about adding weight to your abdominal training.

Nutrition Plan

Continuing what we began last week, this nutrition plan emphasizes consuming only whole, lean foods as your primary source of energy. If you have been incorporating more processed or fattier meats—like turkey bacon, ham, or lean luncheon meats—now is the time to trim those extras. Eat only low-glycemic carbs, like sweet potatoes and oatmeal, and cut out any pasta or breads. Remember, these whole, lean foods are all still good to include in a future healthy diet.

SHOPPING LIST FOR THE WEEK

- For meat: choose from skinless chicken breast, extra-lean ground beef, salmon, canned light tuna
- For vegetarians: choose from tofu, kidney beans
- Foods containing healthy fats: avocados, almonds, edamame beans, fish oil
- Fruit: apples, bananas, blueberries, kiwi
- Hummus
- Low-glycemic carbohydrates: sweet potatoes, wild rice, quinoa, oats
- Omega-3-enriched eggs and carton of egg whites
- PB2 Powdered Peanut Butter
- Protein powder, low-carb
- Low-fat Caesar dressing
- Vegetables: broccoli, green and yellow squash, cauliflower, carrots, celery, bell peppers, romaine lettuce

MEAL PLAN FOR THE WEEK

Breakfast Options

- 1½ scoops protein powder in water with fish oil, and sweet potato hash browns
- 3 whole eggs with oatmeal

Snack Options

- Double serving of vegetables with 4 tablespoons hummus dip

Lunch Options

- Chicken or tofu stir-fry with vegetables over quinoa
- Tuna with wild rice and low-fat Caesar salad

Snack Options

- Egg white omelet with bell peppers and avocado
- 1½ scoops protein powder with PB2 Powdered Peanut Butter and a handful of roasted, salted almonds

Dinner Options

- Extra-lean ground beef or tofu with roasted green and yellow squash and steamed cauliflower
- Salmon over broccoli and carrots or edamame beans with spiraled broccoli stems and bell peppers

Post-Workout Options

- Chicken or tofu with vegetables and sweet potatoes
- Tuna or kidney beans with vegetables and a serving of fruit

DAILY CALORIE, PROTEIN, AND CARB RECOMMENDATIONS

This week, you're following closer to a 40/40/20 macronutrient split, with the majority of your carbohydrates in the first three meals of the day so your body can best use the energy from those foods. Look ahead to Week 9 for more food combinations. Post-workout meals don't always have to be protein shakes, but they should be high in protein and carbs to initiate muscle recovery. See chapter 3 for more suggestions.

Day-by-Day Routines

Focus Legs

Muscles quadriceps, glutes, hamstrings, calves, core muscles (rectus abdominis, internal and external obliques, transverse abdominals, erectors)

Length of Workout 10 to 15 minutes

Repetitions 3 to 5 sets each exercise, 6 to 8 reps

Beginner Workout squats (warm-up), squats (working sets), deadlifts, lunges, wall sits (cool-down)

Intermediate Workout add 3 additional sets of deadlifts with glute bands

Advanced Workout add leg curls

> ### Food TIP
> Keeping up your protein intake throughout the day gives your body the nutrients it needs to repair muscle tissue and develop strength.

Week 8, Day 2

Rest Day

Week 8, Day 3

Focus Shoulders

Muscles deltoids (anterior, medial, posterior), triceps, core muscles (rectus abdominis, internal and external obliques, transverse abdominals, erectors)

Length of Workout 10 to 15 minutes

Repetitions 3 to 5 sets each exercise, 6 to 8 reps

Beginner Workout bent-arm lateral raises (warm-up), shoulder presses, Arnold presses, lying one-arm lateral raises, standing reverse flys (cool-down)

Intermediate Workout add plank walks

Advanced Workout add shoulder press drop-sets

> ## Safety Advice
> Setting up a mirror in your home gym can be a useful tool as you continue to strive for perfect form.

Week 8, Day 4

Focus Back, Core

Muscles latissimus dorsi, rhomboids, trapezius, biceps, core muscles (rectus abdominis, internal and external obliques, transverse abdominals, erectors)

Length of Workout 10 to 15 minutes

Repetitions 3 to 5 sets each exercise, 6 to 8 reps

Beginner Workout Supermans (warm-up), pulldowns, double-grasp rows, V-sit twists, plank walks (cool-down)

Intermediate Workout add leg raises

Advanced Workout add bicycles

> ## Fit TIP
> Breathing correctly during your lifts is better for your health and will improve your strength and ability.

Week 8, Day 5

Rest Day

Week 8, Day 6

Focus Chest, Triceps

Muscles pectorals, anterior deltoids, triceps, core muscles (rectus abdominis, internal and external obliques, transverse abdominals, erectors)

Length of Workout 10 to 15 minutes

Repetitions 3 to 5 sets each exercise, 6 to 8 reps

Beginner Workout push-ups (warm-up), chest presses, tricep push-ups, chest flys, dips (cool-down)

Intermediate Workout add overhead tricep extensions

Advanced Workout add incline presses

> ### Food TIP
> When you're trying to build muscle, you need to eat more calories than you burn during the day. If you're feeling hungry and drinking more water doesn't help, be sure to snack on lean protein and vegetables.

Week 8, Day 7

Focus Biceps, Core

Muscles biceps, core muscles (rectus abdominis, internal and external obliques, transverse abdominals, erectors)

Length of Workout 10 to 15 minutes

Repetitions 3 to 5 sets each exercise, 6 to 8 reps

Beginner Workout bird dogs (warm-up), concentration curls, butterfly crunches, bicycles, planks with shoulder tap (cool-down)

Intermediate Workout add bicep curls

Advanced Workout add pull-ups

> ### Safety Advice
> Of course you are excited to make progress, but listen to your body and don't go too hard, too fast. Injuring yourself by overtraining will not help you reach your fitness goals.

Nutrition Plan

This is an encore of Week 8, a gentle reminder to omit some of your tasty snacks, such as protein bars or natural peanut butter. If you have been finding this hard, a food supplement such as PB2 Powdered Peanut Butter offers a perfect calorie-reduced substitute to satisfy your craving. Eating clean, whole foods will help you build an exceptional physique, and these steps are all preparing you for hitting your peak conditioning in chapter 7.

SHOPPING LIST FOR THIS WEEK

- For meat: choose from skinless chicken breast, extra-lean ground beef, salmon, canned light tuna

- For vegetarians: choose from tofu, kidney beans

- Foods containing healthy fats: avocados, almonds, edamame beans, fish oil

- Fruit: apples, bananas, blueberries, kiwi

- Hummus

- Low-glycemic carbohydrates: sweet potatoes, wild rice, quinoa, oats

- Low-fat Caesar dressing

- Omega-3-enriched eggs and carton of egg whites

- PB2 Powdered Peanut Butter

- Protein powder, low-carb

- Vegetables: broccoli, green and yellow squash, cauliflower, carrots, celery, bell peppers, romaine lettuce

MEAL PLAN FOR THE WEEK

Breakfast Options

- 1½ scoops protein powder in water with fish oil, and sweet potato hash browns

- 3 whole eggs with oatmeal

Snack Option

- Double serving of vegetables with 4 tablespoons hummus dip

Lunch Options

- Chicken or tofu stir-fry with vegetables over quinoa
- Tuna with wild rice and low-fat Caesar salad

Snack Options

- Egg white omelet with bell peppers and avocado
- 1½ scoops protein powder with PB2 Powdered Peanut Butter and a handful of roasted, salted almonds

Dinner Options

- Extra-lean ground beef or tofu with roasted green and yellow squash and steamed cauliflower
- Salmon over broccoli and carrots, or edamame beans with spiraled broccoli stems and bell peppers

Post-Workout Options

- Chicken or tofu with vegetables and sweet potatoes
- Tuna or kidney beans with vegetables and a serving of fruit

DAILY CALORIE, PROTEIN, AND CARB RECOMMENDATIONS

Enjoy your final cheat meal of this transformation after completing your upcoming progress review, to avoid the skewing of your sure-to-be-impressive results by water retention. During the next three weeks, you will be striving to reach a new level of physical fitness rather than maintaining your current physique. This can throw off an otherwise balanced, healthy lifestyle, tilting the scales toward fitness. Your social life may suffer temporarily, but great achievements often require sacrifice.

Day-by-Day Routines

Focus Calves, Core, Glutes

Muscles glutes, quadriceps, calves, core muscles (rectus abdominis, internal and external obliques, transverse abdominals, erectors)

Length of Workout 10 to 15 minutes

Repetitions 3 to 5 sets each exercise, 6 to 8 reps

Beginner Workout bird dogs (warm-up), side-lying hip raises, glute hip thrusts, calf raises, wall sits (cool-down)

Intermediate Workout add butterfly crunches

Advanced Workout add V-sit twists

> ### Fit TIP
> Lower-back pain is a common issue that can be alleviated by strengthening the muscles that surround the spine and support the back.

Week 9, Day 2

Rest Day

Week 9, Day 3

Focus Chest, Shoulders

Muscles pectorals, deltoids, triceps, core muscles (rectus abdominis, internal and external obliques, transverse abdominals, erectors)

Length of Workout 10 to 15 minutes

Repetitions 3 to 5 sets each exercise, 6 to 8 reps

Beginner Workout push-ups (warm-up), shoulder presses, Arnold presses, chest flys, bent-arm lateral raises (cool-down)

Intermediate Workout add shoulder press drop-sets

Advanced Workout add incline presses

> ### Food TIP
> Variety in your food choices will help you cover all the bases when it comes to daily nutrient requirements.

Week 9, Day 4

Focus Arms, Core

Muscles posterior deltoids, biceps, triceps, core muscles (rectus abdominis, internal and external obliques, transverse abdominals, erectors)

Length of Workout 10 to 15 minutes

Repetitions 3 to 5 sets each exercise, 6 to 8 reps

Beginner Workout bird dogs (warm-up), bicep curls, overhead tricep extensions, dips, plank walks (cool-down)

Intermediate Workout add concentration curls

Advanced Workout add push presses

> ### Safety Advice
> Being proactive with recovery methods will greatly reduce your risk of injury, so book yourself a deep-tissue massage, try foam rolling, or soak in a hot bath to ease muscle soreness.

Week 9, Day 5

Rest Day

Focus Hamstrings, Quadriceps

Muscles quadriceps, glutes, hamstrings, calves, core muscles (rectus abdominis, internal and external obliques, transverse abdominals, erectors)

Length of Workout 10 to 15 minutes

Repetitions 3 to 5 sets each exercise, 6 to 8 reps

Beginner Workout squats (warm-up), squats (working sets), lunges, leg curls, wall sits (cool-down)

Intermediate Workout add glute hip thrusts

Advanced Workout add leg abductions

> Fit TIP
> Applying resistance bands around your thighs activates the glutes to correctly engage your muscles during lower-body training.

Focus Back

Muscles latissimus dorsi, rhomboids, trapezius, biceps, core muscles (rectus abdominis, internal and external obliques, transverse abdominals, erectors)

Length of Workout 10 to 15 minutes

Repetitions 3 to 5 sets each exercise, 6 to 8 reps

Beginner Workout Supermans (warm-up), single-arm rows, pulldowns, pullovers, reverse flys (cool-down)

Intermediate Workout add lying one-arm lateral raises

Advanced Workout add straight-arm pushdowns

> ## Food TIP
> Carbohydrates are not the enemy, even when you're trying to get lean. They provide your body's main source of energy and are necessary for muscle development. Not all carbs are created equal! Ideally, choose low-glycemic carbohydrates in your diet, such as brown rice, sweet potatoes, and oats.

> ## Time for a Weigh-In
> You've been crushing your training and have dialed in your eating over the past nine weeks. Ready to see what you've accomplished? Visit page 183 to put another assessment in the books, and prepare yourself for the big changes ahead in the final three weeks.

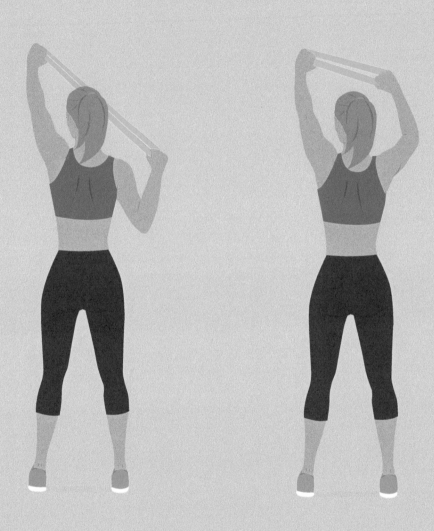

weeks 10 to 12: Hitting your peak

7

You will enjoy this final portion of your workout program as we focus on both boosting your ability and showcasing your hard-earned muscle. The body will respond well to increasing the resistance in every exercise, made possible by demanding fewer repetitions. This alteration to your training style will allow you to max out your power without muscle fatigue. During this last phase, after the first 3 to 5 sets, you want to progressively lower your repetitions from 8 to 2, aiming to safely find your 1-rep-maximum if you have a spotter available to assist you.

Nutrition Plan

Individuals with lower-body fat enjoy more definition in their physiques. The truth is that when you're leaner, your muscles actually look bigger! To cut down over the last weeks, reduce your overall caloric intake by 200 calories per day and continue your intense exercise regimen to aim for a 1-pound weight loss each week. Stop taking a weekly cheat meal until after your 12 weeks is over, to make the most of this final stretch. You should also be doing cardiovascular activities like brisk walking, running, biking, inline skating, or hiking to burn extra calories throughout the week.

SHOPPING LIST FOR THIS WEEK

- For meat: choose from skinless chicken breast, turkey, tilapia, halibut, or other white fish

- For vegetarians: choose from vegetarian meat replacement, tofu, soybeans, tempeh

- Carton of egg whites

- Cinnamon

- Coconut oil

- Foods containing healthy fats: almonds, walnuts, hemp seeds

- Fruit: apples, berries, watermelon, grapes

- Low-glycemic carbohydrates: potatoes, brown rice, oats

- Protein powder, low-carb

- Splenda

- Vegetables: corn, spinach, celery, green beans, asparagus, romaine lettuce, radishes

MEAL PLAN FOR THE WEEK

Breakfast Options

- Oatmeal with sliced almonds and protein powder
- Egg whites with 2 tablespoons hemp seeds and brown rice

Snack Options

- Baked apples with coconut oil, cinnamon, and Splenda
- Berries with small serving of crushed walnuts
- Tilapia or vegetarian meat replacement with leafy greens salad with radishes

Lunch Options (Pre-Workout):

- Turkey or vegetarian meat replacement and asparagus with roasted potatoes
- Halibut or tofu with spinach salad and corn on the cob

Dinner Options

- Soybeans in mixed vegetable stir-fry
- Halibut or tempeh with green beans

Post-Workout Options

- 1 to 2 scoops protein powder mixed in water and a piece of fruit

DAILY CALORIE, PROTEIN, AND CARB RECOMMENDATIONS

You can cut calories without removing carbohydrates. Reducing your fat serving at breakfast by half and eliminating any fats in your afternoon snack achieve the 200 calories-per-day deficit that will create better muscular definition. Cutting out your weekly cheat meal also reduces your food intake to promote fat loss.

Day-by-Day Routines

Focus Glutes or Rest Day

Muscles quadriceps, glutes, hamstrings, calves, core muscles (rectus abdominis, internal and external obliques, transverse abdominals, erectors)

Length of Workout 10 to 15 minutes

Repetitions 3 to 5 sets each exercise, 6 to 8 reps

Beginner Workout squats (warm-up), deadlifts, leg abductions, glute kickbacks, wall sits (cool-down)

Intermediate Workout add 3 working sets of squats

Advanced Workout add 3 working sets of deadlifts

> ### Safety Advice
> A solid core helps with compound lifts such as squats and deadlifts, so be sure to engage your abdominals and keep your back straight during these exercises. Stretch your hamstrings at least three times a week to increase your range of motion and maintain agility.

Focus Core

Muscles rectus abdominis, internal and external obliques, transverse abdominals, erectors

Length of Workout 10 to 15 minutes

Repetitions 3 to 5 sets each exercise, 6 to 8 reps

Beginner Workout bird dogs (warm-up), bicycles, push presses, side planks with torso twist, planks with shoulder tap (cool-down)

Intermediate Workout add push press drop-sets

Advanced Workout add leg raises

> ## Fit TIP
> Try to find support from other fitness-minded individuals who will push you to keep going and help you succeed. Don't let anyone derail you from your goals! Here's some motivation to keep going: You've already reduced your blood pressure, increased oxygen to your muscles, and improved your metabolism through consistent training. It's also likely your skin is brighter and your confidence higher.

Week 10, Day 3

Focus Back, Biceps

Muscles latissimus dorsi, rhomboids, trapezius, biceps, core muscles (rectus abdominis, internal and external obliques, transverse abdominals, erectors)

Length of Workout 10 to 15 minutes

Repetitions 3 to 5 sets each exercise, 6 to 8 reps

Beginner Workout Supermans (warm-up), double-grasp rows, straight-arm pushdowns, concentration curls, standing reverse flys (cool-down)

Intermediate Workout add concentration curl drop-sets

Advanced Workout add bicep curls

> ## Food TIP
> The best way to show off your six-pack abs is to follow a healthy diet and do moderate amounts of cardio before breakfast or post-workout. If you are doing cardio following your workout, move your post-workout meal to after the cardio to maximize the fat-burning potential.

Week 10, Day 4

Rest Day

Week 10, Day 5

Focus Core, Shoulders

Muscles deltoids, triceps, core muscles (rectus abdominis, internal and external obliques, transverse abdominals, erectors)

Length of Workout 10 to 15 minutes

Repetitions 3 to 5 sets each exercise, 6 to 8 reps

Beginner Workout bent-arm lateral raises (warm-up), shoulder presses, lying one-arm lateral raises, butterfly crunches, plank walks (cool-down)

Intermediate Workout add bent-arm lateral raise drop-sets

Advanced Workout add shoulder press drop-sets

> ### Safety Advice
> Keep in mind, your abs and obliques are engaged during compound movements, such as squats, bench and shoulder presses, and deadlifts, and these muscles also need rest days. If your core is still sore, wait another day to lift.

Week 10, Day 6

Focus Legs

Muscles quadriceps, glutes, hamstrings, calves, core muscles (rectus abdominis, internal and external obliques, transverse abdominals, erectors)

Length of Workout 10 to 15 minutes

Repetitions 3 to 5 sets each exercise, 6 to 8 reps

Beginner Workout squats (warm-up), squats (working sets), lunges, leg curls, wall sits (cool-down)

Intermediate Workout add 3 additional sets of lunges

Advanced Workout add 3 additional sets of leg curls

> ### Fit TIP
> If there is an area of your body you are unhappy with, then work every week to strengthen those muscles and you will see improvements! Working on your body includes self-care and proper nutrition, so be proud of yourself for making progress even when you are not lifting.

Focus Chest, Triceps

Muscles pectorals, anterior deltoids, triceps, core muscles (rectus abdominis, internal and external obliques, transverse abdominals, erectors)

Length of Workout 10 to 15 minutes

Repetitions 3 to 5 sets each exercise, 6 to 8 reps

Beginner Workout push-ups (warm up), incline presses, chest flys, tricep push-ups, dips (cool-down)

Intermediate Workout add chest presses

Advanced Workout add overhead tricep extensions

> ### Food TIP
> Keep junk food out of your house if you struggle to stick to the diet so you don't get tempted by the snacks conveniently found in the cupboard. Of course, your family or roommates deserve to enjoy treats and not be subjected to your food choices, but ask them to support your decision to eat better by at least not bringing your biggest temptations and favorite indulgences into the home.

Nutrition Plan

You should still be feeling powerful during your workouts, but to get lean and have deeper cuts in your muscles, dieting to lose body fat is necessary—and somewhat uncomfortable, unfortunately. It's important to overcome fatigue by providing yourself with quality protein and carbohydrates before and after your weight training. Be sure you move your pre- and post-workout meals to when you lift in the day, tapering down your calories as bedtime nears.

SHOPPING LIST FOR THE WEEK

- For meat: choose from skinless chicken breast, turkey, tilapia or halibut or other white fish

- For vegetarians: choose from vegetarian meat replacement, tofu, soybeans, tempeh

- Carton of egg whites

- Cinnamon

- Coconut oil

- Foods containing healthy fats: almonds, walnuts, hemp seeds

- Fruit: apples, berries, watermelon, grapes

- Low-glycemic carbohydrates: potatoes, brown rice, oats

- Protein powder, low-carb

- Splenda

- Vegetables: corn, spinach, celery, green beans, asparagus, romaine lettuce, radishes

MEAL PLAN FOR THE WEEK

Breakfast Options

- Oatmeal with sliced almonds and protein powder

- Egg whites with 2 tablespoons hemp seeds and brown rice

Snack Options

- Baked apples with coconut oil, cinnamon, and Splenda

- Berries with small serving of crushed walnuts

Lunch Options (Best Pre-Workout):

- Turkey or vegetarian meat replacement and asparagus with roasted potatoes

- Halibut or tofu with spinach salad and corn on the cob

Snack Options

- Tilapia or vegetarian meat replacement with leafy greens salad with radishes

Dinner Options

- Soybeans in mixed vegetable stir-fry

- Halibut or tempeh with green beans

Post-Workout Options

- 1 to 2 scoops protein powder mixed in water, and a piece of fruit

DAILY CALORIE, PROTEIN, AND CARB RECOMMENDATIONS

Your macronutrients have been altered to more of a 50/30/20 (protein/carb/fat) split now as you experience a cutting diet for the final weeks of your program. Keeping your protein intake high allows you to promote cell regeneration while decreasing the chance of your body becoming catabolic and tearing down your hard-earned muscle tissue for energy.

Day-by-Day Routines

Focus Legs

Muscles quadriceps, glutes, hamstrings, calves, core muscles (rectus abdominis, internal and external obliques, transverse abdominals, erectors)

Length of Workout 10 to 15 minutes

Repetitions 3 to 5 sets each exercise, 6 to 8 reps

Beginner Workout squats (warm-up), glute hip thrusts, leg curls, calf raises, wall sits (cool-down)

Intermediate Workout add glute kickbacks

Advanced Workout add side-lying hip raises

> ### Safety Advice
> Using a BOSU ball or balance board adds another level of intensity to many exercises and will build a strong core, but the weight used should be reduced when adding this piece of equipment.

Focus Chest, Core

Muscles pectorals, anterior deltoids, triceps, core muscles (rectus abdominis, internal and external obliques, transverse abdominals, erectors)

Length of Workout 10 to 15 minutes

Repetitions 3 to 5 sets each exercise, 6 to 8 reps

Beginner Workout bird dogs (warm-up), chest presses, push presses, side planks with torso twist, dips (cool-down)

Intermediate Workout add 3 additional sets of chest presses

Advanced Workout add chest flys

Week 11, Day 3

Focus Back

Muscles latissimus dorsi, rhomboids, trapezius, biceps, core muscles (rectus abdominis, internal and external obliques, transverse abdominals, erectors)

Length of Workout 10 to 15 minutes

Repetitions 3 to 5 sets each exercise, 6 to 8 reps

Beginner Workout Supermans (warm-up), double-grasp rows, pulldowns, straight-arm pushdowns, standing reverse flys (cool-down)

Intermediate Workout add 3 additional sets of double-grasp rows

Advanced Workout add single-arm rows

> Food TIP
> Sugar cravings are real! To combat an intense need for sweets, get enough sleep, don't skip meals, avoid having desserts as your cheat meal, take a multivitamin, keep busy, stay hydrated, and increase your fiber intake.

Week 11, Day 4

Rest Day

Week 11, Day 5

Focus Legs or Rest Day

Muscles quadriceps, glutes, hamstrings, calves, core muscles (rectus abdominis, internal and external obliques, transverse abdominals, erectors)

Length of Workout 10 to 15 minutes

Repetitions 3 to 5 sets each exercise, 6 to 8 reps

Beginner Workout squats (warm-up), deadlifts, side-lying hip raises, glute kickbacks, wall sits (cool-down)

Intermediate Workout add 3 additional sets of deadlifts

Advanced Workout add lunges

> ### Safety Advice
> Stretching between sets is always a great way to maximize your exercise time, prevent injury by improving agility, and build more attractive muscle belly shapes. Once your hamstrings are more flexible, you may want to elevate yourself on a step during deadlifts, to allow the weight to drop lower for increased range of motion.

Week 11, Day 6

Focus Shoulders

Muscles deltoids, triceps, core muscles (rectus abdominis, internal and external obliques, transverse abdominals, erectors)

Length of Workout 10 to 15 minutes

Repetitions 3 to 5 sets each exercise, 6 to 8 reps

Beginner Workout bent-arm raises (warm-up), shoulder presses, lying one-arm lateral raises, incline presses, standing reverse flys (cool-down)

Intermediate Workout add 3 additional sets of shoulder presses

Advanced Workout add 3 additional sets of reverse flys

> ### Fit TIP
> As your strength improves, you may need to upgrade your home gym to accommodate more challenging exercises. This can include buying heavier dumbbells and investing in a good-quality workout bench so you can safely train with support beyond what a stability ball can provide.

Focus Arms

Muscles anterior and medial deltoids, biceps, triceps, core muscles (rectus abdominis, internal and external obliques, transverse abdominals, erectors)

Length of Workout 10 to 15 minutes

Repetitions 3 to 5 sets each exercise, 6 to 8 reps

Beginner Workout bent-arm lateral raises (warm-up), bicep curls, overhead tricep extensions, concentration curls, plank walks (cool-down)

Intermediate Workout add 3 additional sets of bent-arm lateral raises

Advanced Workout add dips

> ### Food TIP
> If you have a job where you're active, ensure you eat enough carbs to enable your body to build muscle and maintain good brain function. Visit the Resources section at the end of the book to find a helpful, online caloric-intake calculator (see page 185).

Nutrition Plan

If you want to experience a peak week, go to extremes and reduce sodium and fats by cutting back on your salad dressings and diet-friendly sauces. There are also supplements you can purchase to drop water weight if you have a special occasion you want to be ripped for, such as a photo shoot or competition. This week I've added carbs to plump your muscle bellies, give you a fuller look, and empower epic workouts.

SHOPPING LIST FOR THE WEEK

- For meat: choose from canned light tuna, skinless chicken breast, lean steak
- For vegetarians: choose from tofu, tempeh
- Almonds
- Fruit: bananas, honeydew melon, pears, pineapple
- Hummus
- Omega-3-enriched eggs
- Low-glycemic carbohydrates: sweet potatoes, brown rice, oats
- Protein powder, low-carb
- Salsa
- Vegetables: spinach, broccoli, cauliflower, carrots, fennel, cucumbers, snap peas

MEAL PLAN FOR THE WEEK

Breakfast Options:

- 3 eggs with spinach and salsa, and oatmeal

Lunch Option:

- Lean steak or tempeh and large serving of vegetables with brown rice

Snack Options:

- Almonds

- Canned light tuna or hummus on cucumbers

Dinner Option:

- Chicken or tofu with vegetables and sweet potatoes

Post-Workout Option:

- 1 to 2 scoops protein powder mixed in water and a piece of fruit

DAILY CALORIE, PROTEIN, AND CARB RECOMMENDATIONS

Adopting a 40/40/20 (protein/carb/fat) macronutrient breakdown allows space in your diet for dense carbs that will fill up your muscles, ensuring you don't feel flat during your workouts and that you look fantastic for your final assessment photos. Please be sure to share your results with me—I absolutely love to hear client success stories!

Day-by-Day Routines

Focus Core, Legs

Muscles quadriceps, glutes, hamstrings, calves, core muscles (rectus abdominis, internal and external obliques, transverse abdominals, erectors)

Length of Workout 10 to 15 minutes

Repetitions 3 to 5 sets each exercise, 1 to 8 reps

Beginner Workout squats (warm-up), squats (working sets), glute hip thrusts, leg abductions, wall sits (cool-down)

Intermediate Workout add butterfly crunches

Advanced Workout add side planks with torso twist

> ### Safety Advice
> Remember, your body is never the same after an injury, so be open to trying variations on movements but never rush into a new exercise without knowing the correct technique.

Focus Chest, Triceps

Muscles pectorals, anterior deltoids, triceps, core muscles (rectus abdominis, internal and external obliques, transverse abdominals, erectors)

Length of Workout 10 to 15 minutes

Repetitions 3 to 5 sets each exercise, 1 to 8 reps

Beginner Workout push-ups (warm-up), chest presses, chest flys, incline presses, dips (cool-down)

Intermediate Workout add overhead tricep extensions

Advanced Workout add tricep push-ups

> ## Fit TIP
> To show your muscle definition, you need to achieve low levels of body fat. The best time to add fat-burning cardio to your fitness program is either first thing in the morning, before breakfast, or immediately after training, before your post-workout meal.

Week 12, Day 3

Focus Back, Biceps

Muscles latissimus dorsi, rhomboids, trapezius, biceps, core muscles (rectus abdominis, internal and external obliques, transverse abdominals, erectors)

Length of Workout 10 to 15 minutes

Repetitions 3 to 5 sets each exercise, 1 to 8 reps

Beginner Workout Supermans (warm-up), single-arm rows, pull-ups or pulldowns, concentration curls, standing reverse flys (cool-down)

Intermediate Workout add 3 additional sets single-arm rows

Advanced Workout add concentration curl drop-sets

> ## Food TIP
> Never skip breakfast! Eating first thing in the morning boosts energy and focus, keeps your body from becoming catabolic, and will help you feel fuller all day. If you do cardio on an empty stomach in the morning, be sure to eat immediately afterward.

Week 12, Day 4

Rest Day

Week 12, Day 5

Focus Legs or Rest Day

Muscles quadriceps, glutes, hamstrings, calves, core muscles (rectus abdominis, internal and external obliques, transverse abdominals, erectors)

Length of Workout 10 to 15 minutes

Repetitions 3 to 5 sets each exercise, 2 to 8 reps

Beginner Workout squats (warm-up), lunges, glute kickbacks, leg curls, wall sits (cool-down)

Intermediate Workout add 3 additional sets of lunges

Advanced Workout add side-lying hip raises

> ### Safety Advice
> Your body recovers during sleep, so allow yourself at least a good eight hours of rest every night. A well-rested individual looks and feels better all day and is more likely to make healthy food choices. You'll be in a much better mood, too!

Week 12, Day 6

Focus Core, Shoulders

Muscles deltoids, triceps, core muscles (rectus abdominis, internal and external obliques, transverse abdominals, erectors)

Length of Workout 10 to 15 minutes

Repetitions 3 to 5 sets each exercise, 2 to 8 reps

Beginner Workout bird dogs (warm-up), shoulder presses, bent-arm lateral raises, bicycles, standing reverse flys (cool-down)

Intermediate Workout add 3 additional sets of shoulder presses

Advanced Workout add push presses

> ### Fit TIP
> If you have a body part that you want to focus on improving as a priority, try to organize your workout split to train it twice each week. Muscular arms are built during every upper body movement, so isolating biceps and triceps is not always necessary.

Focus Arms

Muscles pectorals, anterior and medial deltoids, biceps, triceps, core muscles (rectus abdominis, internal and external obliques, transverse abdominals, erectors)

Length of Workout 10 to 15 minutes

Repetitions 3 to 5 sets each exercise, 2 to 8 reps

Beginner Workout push-ups (warm-up), Arnold presses, bicep curls, overhead tricep extensions, dips (cool-down)

Intermediate Workout add concentration curls

Advanced Workout add plank walks

Food TIP

Overcome food cravings by drinking water, eating something healthy, chewing sugar-free gum, brushing your teeth, exercising, getting more sleep, stopping boredom, meditating on your goals, eating more fiber—or simply waiting them out!

Time for a Weigh-In

Now that you're in the routine of doing check-ins every three weeks, why stop? This is a great moment to do a final assessment using page 183 to reflect on the changes to your body that 90 days of dedicated training and healthy eating have made possible. You should also commit to continuing to do regular assessments to hold yourself accountable to your fitness goals and benchmark your progress.

PART III

THE EXERCISES

Here's where the magic begins! In the next five chapters, I'll coach you through 40 exercises that will beautifully shape your physique. Each lesson reviews the specific muscle groups involved and provides concise, step-by-step instructions to produce hypertrophy. It lists exercise variations for beginners and modifications for those who are more advanced. And it includes clear illustrations that show how to do each lift perfectly.

To support your fitness transformation, I've got something extra for you! Visit juliegermaine.com/90-day-plan to view video exercise tutorials of each movement. You can also download a free strength chart to record your gains—a useful tool when assessing your results over time.

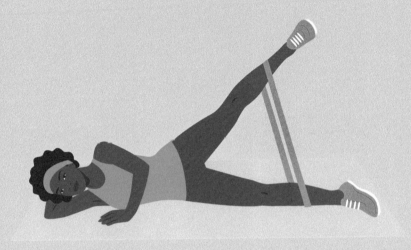

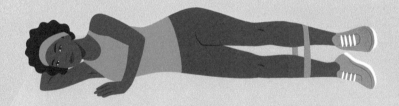

Legs and Glutes

8

In this chapter, you'll learn to love the torture of a sweaty leg day.

Due to the massive size of the leg and glute muscles, these workouts can actually speed up delivery of testosterone and growth hormones to all the muscles. This creates an ideal environment for muscle hypertrophy. So even if you just want to put on size in your upper body, regular leg days are a must.

Training your lower half makes for some of the toughest—and most effective—workouts. Your entire body benefits from a well-organized lower-body weight training session.

warm-up exercise
Squats

Muscles quadriceps, glutes, adductors, erectors, abdominals

Squats are one of the best exercises for the lower body. When you perform exercises that engage your quadriceps, hamstrings, and glutes, your abdominals and back muscles, among others, are often contracted isometrically. For this reason, squats are a perfect warm-up exercise.

INSTRUCTIONS

1. Place a glute band around your thighs. This activates your glutes as you flex your legs to resist the tension. (Whenever you use a glute band, you should "turn out" your thigh muscles, while keeping your toes in the straight-forward position. The knees should never cave inward.)

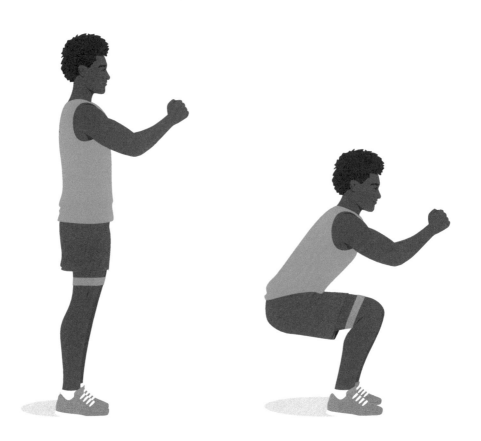

2. Stand with your feet shoulder-width apart, core engaged, and upper body firmly upright. Breathe deeply and hold some air in your chest to set your core to prepare for the movement.

3. While distributing your weight evenly through your heels, push your hips down and "sit back" as you slowly lower your body. Keep your chest up and chin in a neutral position to protect your spine.

4. Lower yourself to a comfortable level based on your flexibility. Having your thighs parallel to the floor is fine, but practice over time should enable you to get your hips lower than your knees without rounding your back.

5. Power through your legs to stand back up again, feeling pressure in your heels.

6. Squeeze your glutes to straighten your body for one count. Then start the next rep.

COMMON MISTAKES AND HOW TO AVOID THEM

Avoid looking down or allowing your upper body to fall forward. It's extremely important that the back remain straight to avoid sudden strain.

REMEMBER

Breathe in as you near the floor and exhale as you exert yourself to stand up. Refrain from fully releasing all the air, to maintain stability in your core while you finish your set.

CHANGE IT UP

If your toes extend past your knees, focus on correcting your form by placing a bench or chair behind you so you feel more comfortable "sitting down" during the exercise. Performing bench squats to sit down with each repetition will help your body get used to the movement.

Grasp dumbbells in each hand to add resistance after your warm-up, to make this exercise a challenge during your working sets. It is most comfortable to rest the weights lightly on your shoulders. Visit juliegermaine.com/90-day-plan to watch a video demonstrating these variations.

Advanced: One option is to stand on an unstable surface, such as a BOSU ball, to fire up your stabilizer muscles. A second option is to explode from the floor with a jump to change your body's response to a bodyweight-only squat.

HIGH-IMPACT EXERCISES
Stiff-Legged Deadlifts

Muscles hamstrings, glutes, erectors, calves

This is my favorite exercise. Deadlifts are a compound movement, which means they incorporate more than one muscle, helping you build strength and muscle quickly. They rely on core strength and stabilize your body to help you with other lifts.

INSTRUCTIONS

1. Place a glute band around your thighs.

2. Stand with your shoulders back, keep your core engaged, and hold two dumbbells in front of your thighs.

3. Bend your knees slightly and lock them in this position for the entire movement.

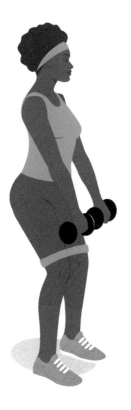
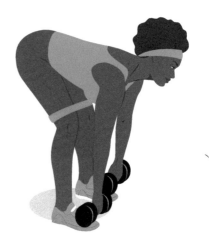

4. Slowly bend at your hip joint, not at your waist, and lower the weights as far as possible while maintaining a straight back. Keeping your eyes forward will help your form. The dumbbells should hang near your legs, basically where your arms naturally fall with gravity. Your hamstring flexibility will affect your range of motion.

5. Squeeze your glutes to begin to pull yourself up slowly. The eccentric motion (with gravity) described in step 4 should take longer than the concentric motion (against gravity) during step 5 to maximize muscle gains.

6. Once you reach your starting position, hold the contraction in your lower body and repeat the exercise for 12 to 15 reps.

7. Rest for 60 seconds, then repeat for 3 sets.

COMMON MISTAKES AND HOW TO AVOID THEM

It's extremely important that your back remain straight and your abdominals remain engaged during the entire exercise. Bending your back can lead to lower-back strain and serious injury.

Performing deadlifts in front of a mirror and holding eye contact when you lower yourself helps keep the back in the correct position. This can put your neck in an unnatural position, so try to look up with your eyes rather than holding your chin too high when you're lowered.

REMEMBER

Tight hamstrings may limit your range of motion and put pressure on your lower back, so incorporating stretches into your fitness program to increase your flexibility will help your muscle development.

CHANGE IT UP

Intermediate: Increasing the weight used for the exercise provides more resistance and amps up difficulty. You can also stand on one leg to challenge your balance and develop your stabilization muscles.

Advanced: Stand on a BOSU ball while performing the exercise.

Lunges

Muscles quadriceps, glutes, hamstrings, calves, core stabilizers

If your goal is to develop your legs and glutes, then lunges are great. They require balance and coordination, and there are many variations that will continue to test your stability and strength. Lunges can also improve your hip flexibility to impact your everyday movement.

INSTRUCTIONS

1. Holding two dumbbells at your sides, stand upright with your feet shoulder-width apart, core and shoulders engaged.

2. Step ahead and lower your hips until your forward leg creates a 90-degree angle. The rear leg should be nearly straight.

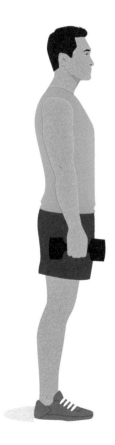
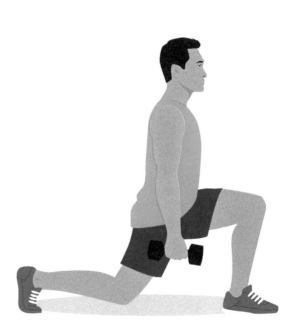

3. Put your weight in your forward heel as you press upward powerfully to step back into the starting position.

4. Repeat this movement with the opposite foot to complete 1 full rep.

COMMON MISTAKES AND HOW TO AVOID THEM

- As you step to lunge, it's almost natural to allow your knee to push forward, but this can lead to repetitive strain injury. To establish proper form, turn sideways to a mirror when you lunge and check that your knee does not extend beyond your toes. Stepping farther out and bending your rear leg more will fix your body positioning.

- Your knees should always be in line with your ankles. Avoid letting them buckle inward.

- Your feet begin shoulder-width apart, and you should maintain that spacing throughout the exercise. If you step forward and minimize this stance (like a tightrope walker), you'll feel off-balance.

REMEMBER

Knee pain is often an indication that your form is not correct.

CHANGE IT UP

If you're a beginner or feel yourself teetering even after fixing the common mistakes, do all the lunges on one side, then switch to the other leg. Pure bodyweight may be an adequate challenge, so add the dumbbells only when ready. In this case, you would start the exercise by stepping forward, feet still shoulder-width apart, bending your legs to a 90-degree angle, and then straightening them without lifting your feet. Don't return to standing with your feet together between each rep. Planting your feet for the duration of each set will help you find your balance and focus on other aspects of the lift until your body becomes steadier.

> **Advanced:** One of my least favorite exercises is the split lunge (also called a split squat), but I do it often because it works extremely well! This more advanced variation requires that you place your back leg on a bench (or chair) for the entire set to further emphasize the force on the forward leg. If you really feel confident, use a stability ball instead of a bench.

Glute Hip Thrusts

Muscles gluteus maximus and medius, hamstrings, quadriceps, adductors, core

Some experts believe that the glute hip thrust is the most effective exercise for building your butt because it maximizes hip extension more than squats or leg presses do. If your fitness goal includes better strength, speed, and power, then don't skip this challenging movement.

INSTRUCTIONS

1. Place a glute band around your thighs.

2. Lay supine (facing up) on a mat on the floor, your feet placed comfortably apart and directly under your knees. If you are performing the exercise with additional weight, such as a dumbbell, this should be pressed on your upper thigh, held in place below your pelvic area.

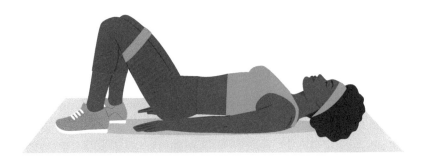

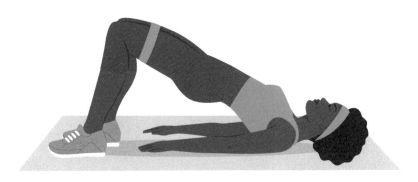

3. Press through your heels and drive your hips upward, squeezing your glutes as far as you can without arching your back.

4. Perform a posterior tilt, which refers to a subtle tilt of your hips upward to "tuck" your butt under.

5. Hold this contraction a moment before slowly lowering your hips until your butt nearly touches the ground.

6. Push back up again to repeat steps 3 to 5, and rest once the recommended rep range is complete.

COMMON MISTAKES AND HOW TO AVOID THEM

If you "feel it" in your lower back rather than your lower body, this simply shows you are weaker in that area. You can also try to slightly adjust the position of your feet until your glutes start to feel more engaged.

REMEMBER

- Keeping your chin tucked in a neutral position can be difficult, but it's as important during this exercise as it is in squats and deadlifts.

- Resist the urge to press through your toes. Your heels should be firmly planted on the ground the entire time.

- Smooth movement will generate the best pump to the muscles. Using momentum is cheating yourself of progress.

CHANGE IT UP

Should you feel too uncomfortable about your form to add weight, you can step things up by pausing at the top of the exercise in a glute bridge for 30 seconds. You can also lift one leg off the ground to try single-leg glute hip thrusts.

> **Advanced:** Elevate your upper body on a bench or resistance ball to increase the range of motion and further activate your core. Place your feet on a stable chair or bench to reverse the elevation and challenge your body in a new way. This version is recommended only as a calisthenic. Visit juliegermaine.com/90-day-plan for video tutorials.

Lying Glute Kickbacks

Muscles gluteus maximus, medius, and minimus

The three parts of the glutes work together as the largest and strongest muscles in the human body and are entirely responsible for the lying glute kickback. This is as close as you can get to a glute isolation exercise, and it will surely lead you to a fuller, rounder butt.

INSTRUCTIONS

1. Lie prone (facing down) on a mat on the floor, in a neutral spine position, and rest your forehead on your hands. For added resistance, place a low-resistance glute band around your ankles. Ankle weights are also effective.

2. With your feet flexed (not pointed) and legs straight, lift one foot up toward the ceiling. Your core remains isometrically contracted to prevent your back from

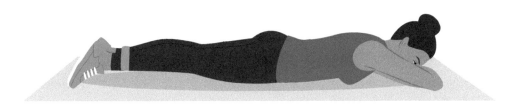

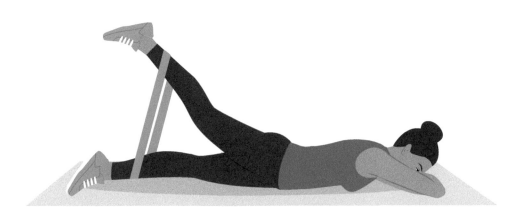

curving during this exercise, and you should feel the burn in your glutes as you push your heel upward.

3. Lower your leg in a controlled motion to tap the floor, then repeat all the reps on one side. Take a brief rest and switch to the other side.

COMMON MISTAKES AND HOW TO AVOID THEM

- It doesn't matter how high you lift your leg; what matters is that you feel your glutes laboring.

- Keeping your upper body somewhat relaxed will ensure your trapezius doesn't tense up. If your shoulders are up to your ears, you become at risk for pulling a muscle in your neck or back.

REMEMBER

Creating a balanced, symmetrical physique promotes a healthy back, so alternate your starting leg to develop strength evenly. If you have already noticed one side being dominant in any unilateral exercise, always begin with your weaker side to stimulate those muscle fibers as a priority.

CHANGE IT UP

Once you're ready for the next challenge, try single-leg glute kickbacks while kneeling on the floor or a bench. Increasing the range of motion and adding an explosive kick intensifies the exercise.

Advanced: A similar exercise that is more challenging is the reverse hyperextension. Lie facedown on a bench with your legs hanging off the end. You could also use a sturdy table or lie over a stability ball with your hands grounded. Your stomach should be as close to the edge of the table as possible while allowing for hip flexion. Hold on securely and squeeze your glutes to raise both legs into the air. Your hips determine the proper range of motion for each rep; your spine and pelvis shouldn't move.

Dumbbell Leg Curls

Muscles hamstrings, glutes, adductors, calves

The hamstrings are the muscle group at the back of the thigh and are underused in everyday life. This can cause a serious imbalance and affect the body's natural function, leading to knee pain and torn tendons. To build strong, robust legs, incorporate isolation exercises to target and grow this muscle group.

INSTRUCTIONS

1. Kneel on a mat on the floor and position a dumbbell upright between your feet so your shoes grip the handles.

2. Lean forward to lie down, head facing the mat to keep the neck in a neutral position. The best position for the arms is hands down beside your body with the elbows up.

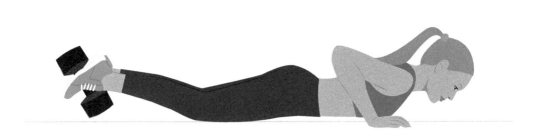

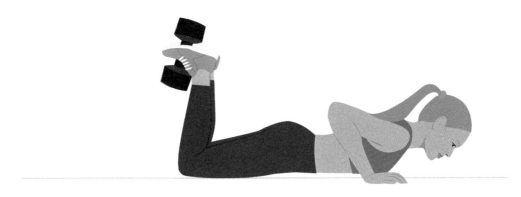

3. Flex your hamstrings to bend your knees and lift the dumbbell up. Try to create a 90-degree angle with your legs, then slowly return the weight to the starting position.

4. Repeat without releasing the tension on the dumbbell until the end of the set.

COMMON MISTAKES AND HOW TO AVOID THEM

- I love doing prone machine leg curls and always recommend my clients use this machine at the gym if possible, but the weight used on this apparatus can be misleading. Start out easy so you can master holding a lighter dumbbell with your feet.

- Point your toes to encourage your entire lower body to engage.

- Your hips should not bend at all. If you feel your glutes rising up, reduce the weight and try again.

REMEMBER

Be confident that you can control the weight you choose. Dropping it midway through your rep is dangerous.

CHANGE IT UP

If your home gym is lacking a dumbbell, try bridge toe taps. Read the glute hip thrusts instructions in this chapter (see page 100) for the starting position. While holding the glute bridge, raise up onto the balls of your feet. Lift one foot and bend your knee to "tap" your toe as close to your glutes as possible. Return the foot to the starting position and switch legs.

You can also isolate your hamstrings with resistance-band leg curls (standing or prone) or perform ball leg curls.

Calf Raises

Muscles gastrocnemius, soleus, tibialis anterior

We are only as strong as our weakest link, right? Well, calves are often that weak link. They tend to be the first muscle of the lower body to fatigue, draining our athletic performance. Calf-specific training not only strengthens the calf muscles but also creates ankle stability, prevents injury, and improves aesthetics.

INSTRUCTIONS

1. Stand on a flat, hard surface with good posture, feet shoulder-width apart. You may want to face a wall so you can place your hands on it for balance.

2. Lean forward as you lift your weight onto the balls of your feet and rise up to your tiptoes.

3. Squeeze your calves and slowly lower your heels back to the floor.

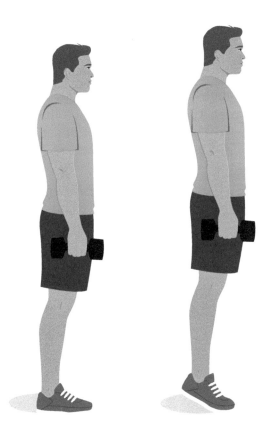

Bouncing during this exercise squanders your energy. This is not the way to build muscle. Your calves will be surprisingly sore if you focus on slowly contracting them and controlling your eccentric and concentric movements. Fighting to keep your balance adds another level of difficulty.

REMEMBER

Fitting in flexibility training will help you maintain an active lifestyle. It feels fantastic to stretch after calf raises in particular. Here's how to isolate your calves for an easy and effective stretch. Stand facing a wall, staying about a foot away from it. Keeping one leg completely straight, bend the other leg and lean into the wall, pushing your weight through the heel of the straight, rear leg. Hold this position for 5 to 15 seconds, then press back to an upright position and repeat for the other calf.

CHANGE IT UP

Adjust your foot position when setting up for this exercise to target the different heads of the gastrocnemius. Turn out your legs from your hips so your toes point away from each other to emphasize the lateral head. Point your toes inward to focus on building up the medial head. I often create workout programs for clients that prescribe sets of 15: 5 reps with toes forward, 5 reps with toes facing out, and 5 reps with toes facing in.

> **Advanced:** Grab a dumbbell to practice progressive overload with this exercise. Stand on the bottom step of your stairs or an aerobic step with your heel hanging off the edge. Hold the weight in one hand and stabilize yourself with the other. Allow your body to lower until you feel a stretch in the calf, then press through the ball of your foot to raise to your tiptoes. Ensure your shoes have good grips to prevent slipping.

Leg Abductions

Muscles gluteus medius and minimus, tensor fasciae latae

To strengthen the glutes and improve your coordination and stability, your fitness program must include a variety of natural movements that work the leg's full function. Though you don't sidestep often, mimicking this ability during your strength training recruits and builds new butt muscles.

INSTRUCTIONS

1. Lie on your side on a mat on the floor, legs straight with a low-resistance glute band around your ankles. Rest your head on one arm in a comfortable position. Balance your body by placing your other arm on the floor in front of you.

2. Lift your upper leg toward the ceiling, being mindful of the position of your trunk. Your abs should be engaged and your back should remain in a straight, neutral position. Your toes should point forward and your leg should not rotate.

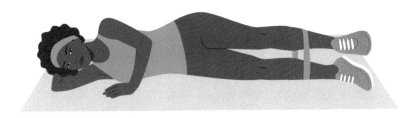

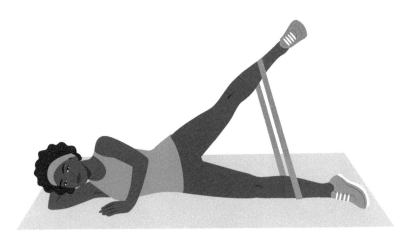

3. Pause to intensify the exercise and then slowly drop your leg until just before it touches the lower leg.

4. Complete your specified number of reps before resting. Repeat on the other side.

COMMON MISTAKES AND HOW TO AVOID THEM
Even though this exercise is done one leg at a time, you're actually working both sides of your body every time. To match the effort applied to each leg, you do need to switch sides and complete equal repetitions per side, but take a rest between every set.

REMEMBER
Despite the fact that you're not moving a lot of weight, paying close attention to your form on abduction exercises is always valuable. You will get the most from your training sessions if you always consider the intent of an action and execute it perfectly.

CHANGE IT UP
Stand up and perform this exercise while holding onto something for stability. If you have a good set of exercise bands, you should be able to keep sufficient resistance by using them. You can also hold a plate, dumbbell, or other heavy object gently against the outer thigh of the working leg.

> **Advanced:** Once your body has adjusted and you feel grounded and secure lifting one leg laterally, you can begin to add movements. Option 1: Squat between each standing-leg abduction and alternate sides for longer sets. Option 2: Move across the floor by taking exaggerated steps sideways with each lateral leg raise. Rest, then repeat while moving in the opposite direction.

Side-Lying Hip Raises

Muscles gluteus medius and minimus, tensor fasciae latae

Here's an exercise that implements movement you don't use often in daily life, unless you are a hockey player or ballet dancer. This simple yet effective action will define your butt and create that glute "shelf" to emphasize fullness. Your core and upper body also get a workout as you strive for balance.

INSTRUCTIONS

1. Place a glute band around your thighs just above your knees. Lie on your side on a mat, your legs bent, leaning into your straight supporting arm.

2. Open your knees to lift your upper leg, thinking about applying force through your grounded knee. At the same time, raise your upper body by pressing your hips forward. Your hip flexibility establishes how open your legs are at the finish.

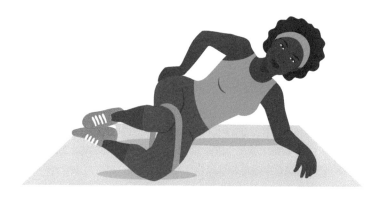

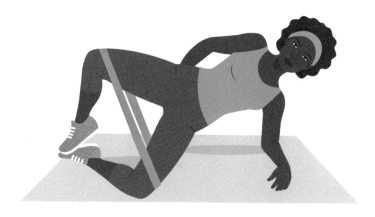

3. Slowly sink back into the starting position, but resist a full relaxation of the muscles until you have done your entire set.

4. Turn over and repeat on the other side.

COMMON MISTAKES AND HOW TO AVOID THEM
- You can elevate yourself by using a pad under your knee in addition to the mat if you are uncomfortable or want to increase the range of motion.

- Keep your head and neck in neutral alignment.

REMEMBER

This exercise is effective and appropriate for both men and women. To build a complete, strong physique with lower-body definition, men also need to train their hip muscles. Having stability in your thighs will allow you to achieve bigger lifts in exercises like squats, deadlifts, and lunges. By isolating underused areas in your body, you strengthen it as a whole.

CHANGE IT UP

This exercise is a more advanced version of the clam, in which you remain on the floor and open your knees without raising your hips off the ground. It's completely fine to start with that and progress as your body adapts.

Advanced: Add difficulty by squeezing and holding at the peak and drawing out the eccentric movement. You can also use a high-resistance band. Your body needs to be compelled to change constantly—don't let yourself get too comfortable or you'll risk hitting a plateau and stop advancing.

COOL-DOWN EXERCISE
Wall Sits

Muscles quadriceps, glutes, calves

This exercise is ideal when you are training outside because it requires no equipment and can be a fun, competitive challenge between workout buddies. Holding a legitimate wall sit takes mental determination, fantastic physical endurance, and exceptional muscle strength. The isometric contraction of your leg muscles expands your body's capabilities.

INSTRUCTIONS

1. Stand with your back firmly pressed against the wall, glute band around your upper thighs to further engage your lower body.

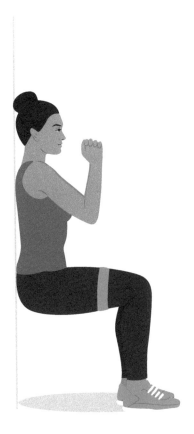

2. Flex your thighs and "turn out" your legs from the hips while keeping your toes forward to activate all your lower-body muscles.

3. Slide down the wall to create a 90-degree angle with your legs. Your feet should be about shoulder-width apart and your knees shouldn't reach beyond the toes.

4. Squeeze! As you push through your heels into the ground, your lower body and core should be tense. Your current fitness level will determine the duration of your set.

5. Stand up to rest, then repeat for the desired number of sets.

> ### Fit TIP
> Your rest period is an opportune time to stretch out your body and prepare it for the next set.

COMMON MISTAKES AND HOW TO AVOID THEM

Although they can appear easy, wall sits are actually quite a difficult exercise. Your mind-body connection is more important than ever to reap the benefits and not agitate your knees. Holding a firm contraction throughout the exercise will guarantee your muscles do the work to cement you in place safely.

REMEMBER

Everyone begins at a different place, so if this exercise is a hard one for you, stay positive and keep at it. You can gradually improve your endurance by starting the wall sit from a higher position and without the glute band.

CHANGE IT UP

Try doing single-leg extensions during the wall sit. I recommend starting with 6 to 8 per side, then continue to hold your wall sit to failure.

Incorporate your stability ball into this movement to further cultivate your balance. Place the ball behind your back, between yourself and the wall, then follow steps 2 through 5 above.

Advanced: Multitask your workouts by incorporating wall sits into other workout days. For example, you can hold a wall sit while performing bicep curls, shoulder presses, or front raises.

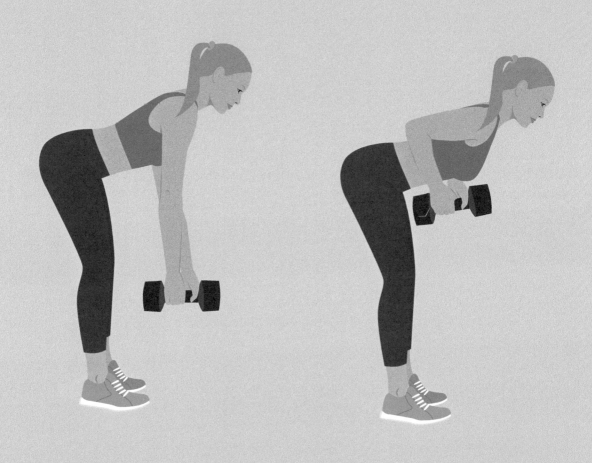

9

Back

Building a strong, wide back has many benefits. You will look better from improved posture, and you will appear to have a smaller waist. An impressive back will also enable you to put on more overall body mass while protecting your spine. As you strengthen your back, keep in mind that it is important to balance the muscle development by working on the front of your body, such as your pecs.

warm-up exercise
Supermans

Muscles erector spinae, glutes, hamstrings

Warming up your body before training is extremely important and should never be skipped. Protecting your spine by strengthening it through subtle movements will improve your athletic performance and help you continue to be active and pain-free for a long time.

INSTRUCTIONS

1. Lie facedown on a mat with your arms stretched out overhead, palms facing each other and your legs straight and parted comfortably.

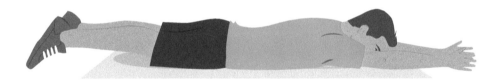

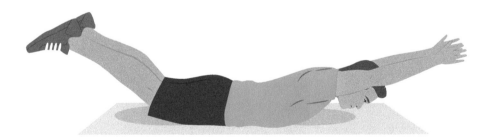

2. Simultaneously raise your upper body and your lower body by contracting your upper back and glutes. Your head should naturally lift as well. Abdominals and lower-back muscles work to stabilize the trunk.

3. Exhale as you lift, and inhale slowly as you lower yourself back to the mat (see step 1).

COMMON MISTAKES AND HOW TO AVOID THEM

- Though this exercise is called "Superman" because it appears as though you are trying to take off from the ground and fly, you should not attempt to launch yourself from the floor in a jerking motion. Careful and disciplined execution will be far more productive.

- Your arms should extend overhead, forming a Y with your body, not a T. The latter would put unwanted pressure on your shoulder joints.

- Exhaling fully and starting from a relaxed position between each rep is denying yourself the satisfaction of a job well done! You should always keep the muscles being worked under pressure until the set is over. Regain your composure and catch your breath during your rest, then endure the pain from lactic acid build-up once again.

REMEMBER

This exercise is a nice warm-up but can also be incorporated into future workouts as a superset to other compound back or glute movements. A superset is when you complete one exercise, then immediately do a second exercise without resting. This training technique works by pushing the muscle closer to failure with each extended set, demanding that serious repair be done to strengthen muscle tissues, resulting in fast gains.

CHANGE IT UP

No equipment is needed for this to be a challenge for most people. You can pause in "flight mode" to push your endurance and promote muscle generation.

Try adding a light glute band around your forearms to step up the difficulty.

> **Advanced:** Adding ankle weights and light dumbbells held in each hand would make you a true superhero in my eyes.

HIGH-Impact Exercise
Single-Arm Band Pulldowns

Muscles latissimus dorsi, teres major, biceps

This variation of the bodybuilding gym exercise cable lat pulldowns is one I use often during my home workouts. My preference is to do one arm at a time, but if you own a longer resistance band and want to wrap it above to do both arms together, that is also acceptable.

INSTRUCTIONS

1. Stand upright, one arm straight overhead holding one end of the band securely. This arm will not move during the exercise.

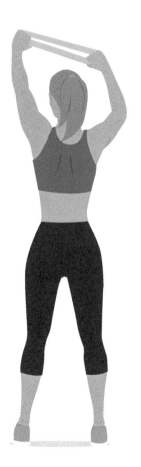 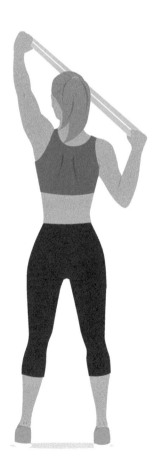

2. Reach up with the other arm and grasp the other end of the band. Focus on pulling your elbow down to the side to form a 90-degree angle, like drawing back on a bow and arrow if you were shooting it up into the sky. You can lower your elbow slightly farther back to increase the range of motion, but it should pull out and away from the body rather than down alongside it.

3. Slowly return the arm to the starting position and complete all reps, then repeat the exercise on the other side.

COMMON MISTAKES AND HOW TO AVOID THEM

- Keep your body open throughout the exercise and avoid letting your shoulders round forward. Imagine a rope being pulled from the center of your chest up toward the ceiling to help you force good posture and avoid sinking down with the movement of your arm.

- The back is a tough area to target for many people. Look at a diagram of the human body to better understand the muscles involved in these exercises and help you connect with what you should be feeling.

REMEMBER

Whenever exercising with resistance bands, safety is always a concern, but this is especially crucial with movements that direct the band toward your face. Be 100 percent certain that your tubing or band is secure when you wrap it around an object or use your body to hold it in place. Serious injury, such as the loss of an eye, can occur if your equipment suddenly snaps free and recoils into your body.

Your grip strength and forearms also benefit from back training.

CHANGE IT UP

Upgrade to the next resistance band level as your body grows stronger week by week. You can also pause when the body is flexed to incorporate isometric contraction and encourage muscle hypertrophy. Visit my website for guidance on great-quality sets of bands.

Double-Grasp Rows

Muscles rhomboids, trapezius, latissimus dorsi, infraspinatus, posterior deltoid, biceps

When training at home as opposed to at a fitness facility, you need to learn how to re-create machine exercises with limited equipment. This take on the seated cable row can be accomplished using a dumbbell or a heavy household object.

INSTRUCTIONS

1. Stand with your feet slightly wider than shoulder-width apart, upper body held in an engaged, stable position. The dumbbell you are using should be on the floor in front of you.

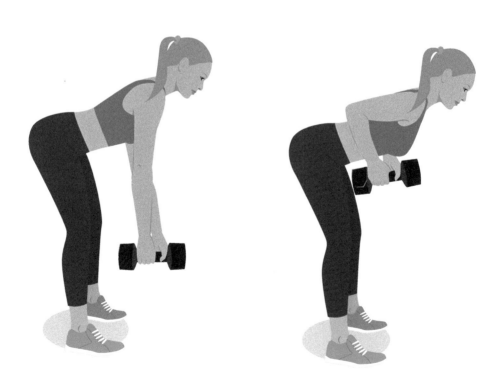

2. Squat down and bend at the hips, without rounding your lower back, and use both hands to firmly grasp the dumbbell. If using another heavy object instead of a dumbbell, make sure you have a firm grip on the weight.

3. Maintaining the bent-over position with a straight back, use your legs to lift the weight off the ground. This is your starting position.

4. Use your back to pull the weight into your stomach. Anchor it there for a short time, then slowly release your muscles to return it to the starting position.

5. Repeat for the specified number of reps, then squat down to return the weight safely to the floor before resting.

COMMON MISTAKES AND HOW TO AVOID THEM

You must lift with your legs and not your back, even with seemingly light objects. Developing this good habit will serve you well in all areas of your life. Lower-back pain and injury is far too common, and everyone is at risk for such a strain.

REMEMBER

Underestimate the weight you should use and build up the resistance set by set, rather than grabbing a heavy weight for the first set. You can always hold the contraction a little longer to be sure every rep has an impact, rather than risk injury.

CHANGE IT UP

This exercise can be performed with a glute band. Place one foot on each end of the band and grasp the middle of the band with both hands.

Advanced: If you feel you've mastered activating the muscles of the back, you can start to isolate them to get more out of every exercise. In the double grasp-row, you can increase your range of motion and engage the infraspinatus, latissimus dorsi, and posterior deltoids by allowing your shoulders to move slightly forward, getting deeper into the stretch when the weight is lowered to the floor. You then retract the shoulders before lifting the weight. As with every exercise in this book, please visit juliegermaine.com/90-day-plan to watch video tutorials that will help you perfect your form and understand the advanced variations.

Pullovers

Muscles latissimus dorsi, serratus anterior, pectoralis major, triceps brachii long head, teres major

Hitting all the muscles in the back while training at home with limited equipment can be difficult, but not impossible. This exercise will widen your back and produce the illusion of a smaller waist as a result.

INSTRUCTIONS

1. Lie with your feet firmly planted on the floor and your back on a stability ball or bench. Hold a dumbbell with both hands so the handle is perpendicular to the floor, and lift it to the starting position above your head, arms extended but elbows not locked straight. You can substitute the type of weight if a dumbbell is not available, but it must be an object that you have a good grasp on because it will be raised over your face.

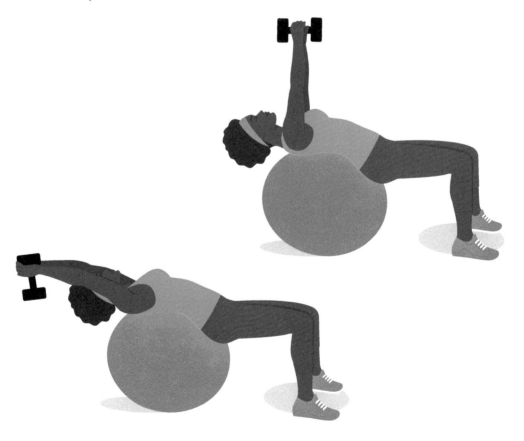

2. Breathe in as you lower the dumbbell behind your head, arms firm in a nearly straight (but not locked) position. Keep your abs contracted to prevent your back from arching.

3. Exhale and pull the weight back up to the starting position with your arms extended toward the ceiling.

COMMON MISTAKES AND HOW TO AVOID THEM

- This exercise puts the shoulder joints in a susceptible position. Lower the weight only until your hands are at about the same level as your head, which can be difficult to gauge if you're training alone. You should feel a stretch through your latissimus dorsi and have no pain in your shoulders.

- Your body responds best to slower, focused movements.

REMEMBER

Begin with a light weight to get used to the exercise before graduating to heavier resistance. The last thing you want is to jump into lifting heavy and dislocate your shoulder.

CHANGE IT UP

You can re-create this action in a standing position using a band. Hold the band in one hand that is extended above you. Grip the other end of the band with the hand of the working side, palm facing down, and press the working arm down toward the body. Your shoulders should be back and your core tight throughout. Squeeze to hold the contraction when your arm is at eye level and then gently raise the arm back up to the starting position.

Straight-Arm Pushdowns

Muscles latissimus dorsi, serratus anterior, pectoralis major, triceps brachii long head, teres major

Here's another unique back move to develop thickness and fullness. This is an alternative to pullovers that uses only a band and works your latissimus dorsi in the lower range of motion. Building your back using variety in movement to keep your body guessing is always good.

INSTRUCTIONS

1. Hold the band in one hand with your straight arm raised out in front of you and at a 45-degree angle toward the ceiling.

2. Grip the other end of the band with the hand of the working side, palm facing down. Your shoulders should be held back and your core tight throughout this exercise.

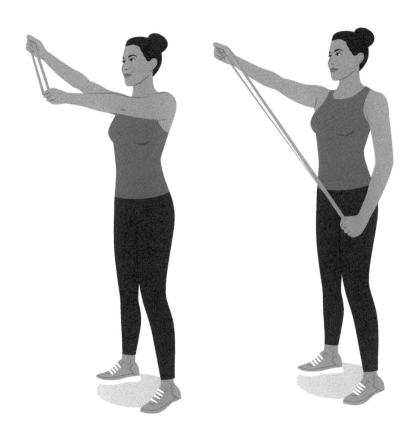

3. Press the working arm down toward the body until it is straight at your side, keeping the other arm frozen as an anchor against pressure.

4. Squeeze your back and hold this position for a few seconds.

5. Slowly return your arm forward and up to the first angle. Your working arm should now be parallel to the floor.

6. Repeat for the specified number of reps before releasing the tension on your band.

COMMON MISTAKES AND HOW TO AVOID THEM

- In order to create an impressive V-taper shape in your back, you need to incorporate full range of motion. Your back should bear resistance as you move your working arm from about eye level down to your side.

- Be wary of your setup and have a good grip on your band. It's very painful when a resistance band slides free and slaps back at you or your workout partner. Serious, permanent injuries can occur.

REMEMBER

- Your chest should remain up and open during this exercise. You will feel your rib cage lift slightly at the full contraction, indicating your back is properly engaged.

- Try to squeeze your shoulder blades together at the very end of the exercise. Making this mind-muscle connection improves fitness results.

- Exhale as you push down, and inhale as you raise your arm.

CHANGE IT UP

This exercise can be replaced with pullovers (see page 122) if you prefer more of a stretch in the latissimus dorsi. Never overextend the shoulder joint.

Pushdowns using tubing are an option, but I avoid this piece of exercise equipment due to the high risk of accidents that can occur with improper setup. Some people who exercise at home create anchors that allow them to hook the tubing around the top of their closed doorways, but if this goes wrong, a tube retracting with force against your body is extremely dangerous.

Pull-Ups

Muscles trapezius, latissimus dorsi, teres major, biceps

There's no reason you can't take your training outdoors, weather permitting! To keep things interesting and fun, I recommend finding a park or a playground and using the structures during your workout. Pull-ups are a challenging exercise that will strengthen and broaden your back.

INSTRUCTIONS

1. Reach up to the monkey bars and take a wide grip.

2. Inhale a deep breath. Exhale as you use your back and arms to lift your body and bring your chest as close to the bar as you can.

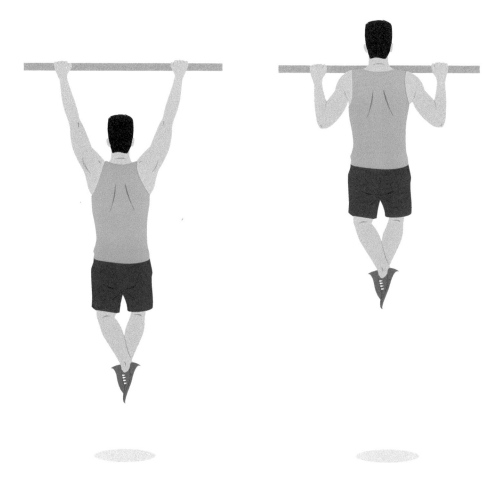

3. Slowly lower yourself back down to hang under the bar.

4. Repeat for your specified number of reps.

COMMON MISTAKES AND HOW TO AVOID THEM
If you lack the strength to do this exercise, try jumping up to the bars or having a workout partner support some of your weight as you lift yourself up, and then fight against gravity to lower yourself down slowly on your own. The eccentric portion of every exercise is when the most strength can be gained, so even if you need help getting up to the bar, this exercise can benefit you.

REMEMBER

There is conflicting advice on the proper way to breathe during this movement. My recommendation is to exhale on exertion, in this case when you pull up. Inhale as you lower yourself down.

CHANGE IT UP

- Chin-ups (pull-ups with your hands closer together, grasping the bar in an underhand grip) are easier to do. This variation also puts more emphasis on the biceps.

- If you aren't able to get outside to do pull-ups, replace these sets in your workout with pulldowns using a band (see page 118).

Single-Arm Dumbbell Rows

Muscles rhomboid major, trapezius, latissimus dorsi, posterior deltoid, biceps

This excellent compound exercise targets the back, shoulders, biceps, and core. If you're limited on time, exercises like this that combine multiple body parts into one workout session will help you train your full body over the week. The row movement is easy to master, and adapting it for the home is possible even if you don't have dumbbells.

INSTRUCTIONS

1. Find a bench, stable chair, or countertop to lean on with one arm as a support. You can also stagger your stance, bend your knees slightly, and place a hand on your thigh to use your leg as the foundation.

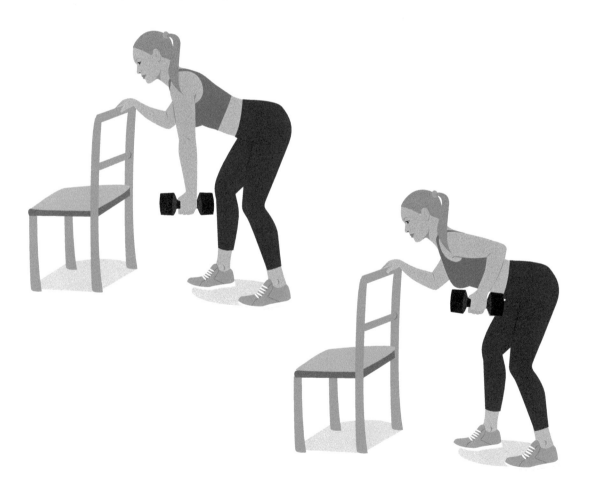

2. Hold a dumbbell in your free hand.

3. Establish good posture in your body (shoulders back, neck in neutral position, core engaged) and maintain this form while you bend at the hips to bring your upper body to a 90-degree angle to the floor.

4. Allow your working arm to hang and then focus on squeezing your back to lift the dumbbell up to your stomach. Your bending arm should slide against your body as it travels up toward your stomach.

5. Hold the contraction briefly.

6. Lower the weight deliberately to further fatigue the muscles.

COMMON MISTAKES AND HOW TO AVOID THEM
Your back should be straight from the start with no twisting or arching.

REMEMBER
Rows will create a wider, thicker back that can help enhance symmetry in your physique and improve your quality of life. This area of the body is often overlooked and under-trained, causing poor posture and back pain.

CHANGE IT UP
Loop a resistance band around your left foot and stand firmly with this leg forward. Grab the band with your right hand and lean over into the starting position (chest parallel to the ground), then pull back your arm to bring the band up and against your body. Tense and pause, then gradually return to the beginning position.

This exercise can be used as a primary muscle builder near the beginning of your workout or as a superset to another compound exercise.

It can also be used in your shoulder workout if you change the angle of your elbow to pull laterally upward so that the band doesn't touch your body as you exert yourself. This slight adjustment puts more focus on the posterior deltoid and is referred to as face pulls. Again, ensure that the band is secure under your feet.

COOL-DOWN EXERCISE
Standing Reverse Flys

Muscles infraspinatus, trapezius, teres minor, posterior deltoids

This is another favorite exercise, which I credit for the definition in my delts and back. If you want nice, rounded shoulders to show off, then becoming a pro with standing reverse flys will help you achieve your goal.

INSTRUCTIONS

1. Stand with your feet apart in a balanced position, holding a dumbbell (or other heavy object) in each hand. Roll your shoulders back to safely prepare your upper body and midsection.

2. Bend at your hips to bring your upper body parallel to the floor, back straight. Your arms naturally fall downward and should have a slight bend in them.

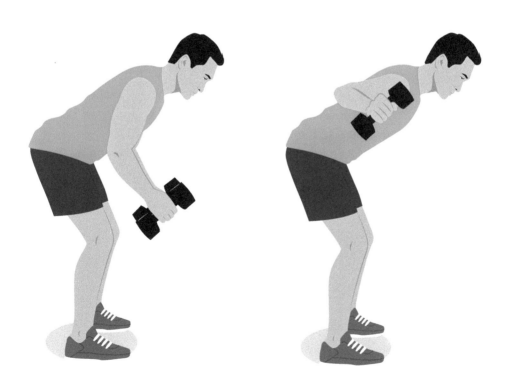

3. Engage your back and rear shoulder muscles to raise the dumbbells out to the sides in alignment with your upper body. Your arms don't bend farther to perform this action but remain locked in the starting position.

4. Slowly resist gravity as you return the weights to the starting position, touching each other.

5. Complete the specified repetitions and carefully pull yourself up to a standing position without rounding your back.

COMMON MISTAKES AND HOW TO AVOID THEM

- Don't allow your shoulders to fall forward when you lean into the starting position. The strong, good posture you have when standing should translate into the exercise for the entire movement.

- Swinging the weight a bit to get it into the raised position isn't wrong. If you try to do this exercise too slowly, you'll put more tension on your neck.

REMEMBER

You're aiming to lift the weights sideways to the height of your body. Don't overextend and raise them higher than that.

CHANGE IT UP

More weight will lead to better results! If you don't have the equipment available to lift heavier, try a drop-set to fully fatigue the muscle bellies.

To perform this exercise using bands, stand upright and hold the band with two hands, arms straight out in front of you at eye level with a slight bend in your elbows. Contract your back and delts to stretch the band as your hands move away from each other horizontally, and then slowly return to starting position. There is no need to bend over when using glute bands in this movement.

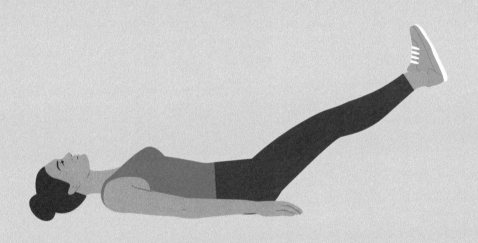

10

abs

Having a six-pack is the motivation for many people to train their abs, but the real reason you should incorporate core isolation is to strengthen the muscles that protect your spine.

warm-up exercise
Core Activation and Bird Dogs

Muscles erector spinae, rectus abdominis, transverse abdominals, glutes

Learning how to move your arms and legs while maintaining a properly engaged core helps prevent back injury. This exercise helps you build the strength to stabilize your entire body, preparing you to use the technique to move with complete confidence and control.

INSTRUCTIONS

1. Core activation: kneel on a mat on all fours—knees under hips, hands under shoulders.

2. Exhale deeply while drawing your abs in toward your spine to learn how to activate the transverse abdominals.

3. Continue to breathe while holding your tummy in. If you feel the sensation of your abs being engaged, great job! Getting the internal core muscles to fire up causes all the other muscles to jolt into action tightly around them. To firm your body up one more level, ever so slightly roll your shoulder blades back and squeeze them together.

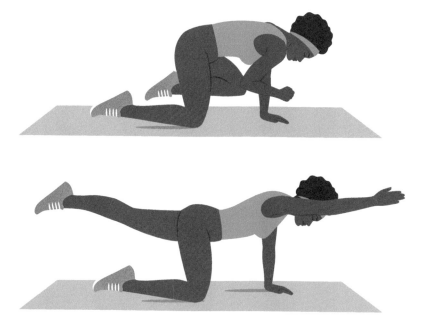

4. Practice this hold and then progress to a plank (see Change It Up) until you feel comfortable adding movement before attempting the bird dog.

5. Bird dogs: From the kneeling position, with your core engaged, raise your right arm and left leg keeping your torso perfectly straight and parallel to the floor.

6. Your right arm and left leg should both end up straight. Imagine yourself lengthening from your fingertips through your heel while you hold the pose.

7. Lower your limbs and squeeze your obliques to gently touch your right elbow to your left knee under your body, then begin your second repetition as you extend back to the open position (step 6).

8. Lower yourself to the first kneeling position and then repeat for the left arm and right leg.

9. Repeat for an equal number of reps per side.

COMMON MISTAKES AND HOW TO AVOID THEM

There are variations of the bird dog that activate the obliques to twist the body upward, but you should develop your form in the standard exercise before moving on to those.

REMEMBER

- To maintain a neutral spine during this simple core exercise, engage your abdominal muscles from the beginning to the end. Focus your brain on the end result—core stability—so you don't get concerned about how high your extremities raise.

- Use this skill of engaging your core in every fitness opportunity, even during a calf or arm exercise.

CHANGE IT UP

To do a plank, engage your core as described in steps 1 to 3, then lower yourself down on your forearms and extend your legs straight back to balance on your toes. This exercise builds a wonderful foundation of core strength.

> **Advanced:** Hold the extended position and pulse the leg and arm up and down in small movements.

High-Impact Exercise
Push Presses

Muscles rectus abdominis, anterior deltoids

The abdominals react to resistance training the same way as every other muscle in the body. Progressively overloading the area by increasing the weight used during exercise will cause the muscle to repair stronger and fuller. This straightforward core exercise is simply amazing for developing the six-pack muscles.

INSTRUCTIONS

1. Lie back on a mat and engage your core, feeling the midsection compress toward your spine.

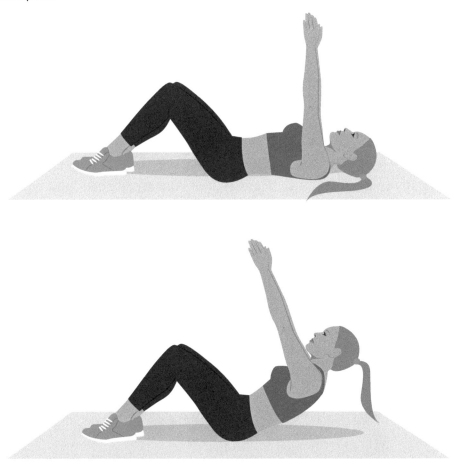

2. Hold this corset-like contraction and lift your shoulders off the ground while reaching upward with your arms.

3. Freeze and squeeze, then do the reverse to complete the rep.

You don't need to do a full sit-up to capitalize on the benefits of abdominal exercises. The subtle movement of getting your shoulder blades off the ground is a sufficient range of motion. Your hip flexors actually take over to pull the body to a sitting position, so don't jerk yourself all the way up. Doing so may put unnecessary strain on your neck and keep you from completing your workout due to soreness.

REMEMBER

- Exhale as you crunch up, and keep breathing while you hold. Learning to control your respiratory system while exercising will make your workouts more enjoyable and productive.

- Your arms don't need to bend, but if you want to incorporate your pecs and triceps into the exercise, you can begin with a dumbbell, medicine ball, or other heavy object held against your chest, and simultaneously perform the abdominal crunch while extending your arms to press the weight up to the ceiling.

CHANGE IT UP

Grab a weight and hold it with both hands above your chest. "Push" it toward the ceiling with each rep to add difficulty to the movement.

Use a stability ball to force your abs to stabilize your body during the movement and to increase your range of motion as you arch back over the ball on the descent. Advanced exercisers can try a combination pullover/push press on the ball. Visit juliegermaine.com/90-day-plan for video tutorials.

Side Planks with Torso Twist

Muscles abdominal muscles, deltoids

All planks serve to improve physical endurance and develop core stability, but this dynamic plank will take your fitness—and your abdominal definition—to a new level. Twisting side planks recruit the total body, which means more bang for your buck! In this exercise the upper and lower body fight for balance while the obliques are engaged in an entirely unique way.

INSTRUCTIONS

1. Get into position on your side on a mat by balancing on one forearm and the edge of your foot. Engage your core and keep your chin at a neutral angle.

2. Straighten your upper arm to point at the ceiling.

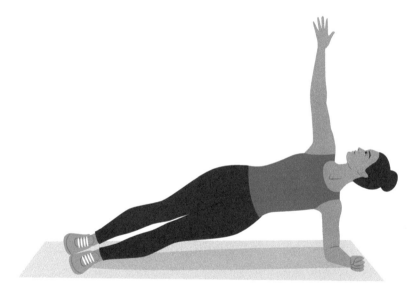

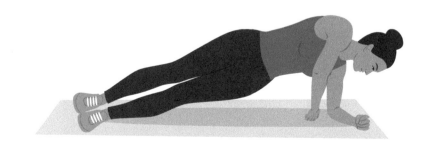

3. Bend your arm to touch the same shoulder, and then twist your torso to bring your elbow to graze the floor.

4. Execute these steps in reverse to complete the first repetition.

5. After completing the specified number of reps, take a short break to catch your breath, and repeat on the other side. Always do the same number of reps on each side of your body.

COMMON MISTAKES AND HOW TO AVOID THEM

Maintaining a neutral spine is important at all times. Imagine you have an egg tucked gently under your chin. Lift your head and the egg will fall, but press your chin down and the egg will crack. Keeping that natural spacing protects you against back injury.

REMEMBER

Your pelvis should not tilt back during isometric exercises like front planks, and the same is true when variations of exercises are performed. Weak abdominal muscles can cause anterior hip tilt, so be sure your neutral spine carries down through the lower body to alleviate back pain.

CHANGE IT UP

Advanced: You can alternate from one side to the other if you have great stamina. Complete a twisting plank with your left side touching the ground, but instead of tapping your right elbow on the floor, plant the forearm down to transition into a front plank. Then continue to follow your momentum by pushing off the floor with your left hand and doing a right-side plank. Finish the movement by raising your left arm into the air. Repeat this up-and-down action for the desired number of reps.

Leg Raises

Muscles hip flexors (iliopsoas pectineus, sartorius, adductor longus, tensor fasciae latae), abdominals (rectus abdominis, external obliques)

Leg raises unify the abdominal muscles to isometrically stabilize your body while also strengthening the anterior hip flexors. This exercise puts emphasis on the rectus abdominis near the pelvis region and is a great addition to a well-rounded core training program.

INSTRUCTIONS

1. Lie flat on your back on a mat with your arms relaxed at your sides. Breathe out and engage your core.

2. Keeping your back flat, slowly raise your legs toward the ceiling until they are perpendicular to the floor.

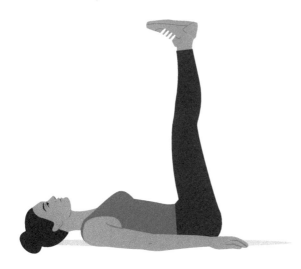

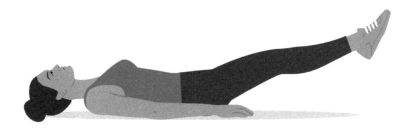

3. Inhale and lower your legs, resisting gravity, until your heels are hovering just above the mat. This is 1 rep.

4. Without resting, begin your second rep.

COMMON MISTAKES AND HOW TO AVOID THEM

- You're primarily working the hip flexors, but the transverse abdominals and rectus abdominis also contract tightly during this exercise.

- If your abs are not strong enough to keep your lower back firmly pressed against the ground, decrease the difficulty of the movement by lowering only one leg at a time. Your starting position would be with both legs pointed straight up in the air.

REMEMBER

Exercises are sometimes referred to as targeting the "lower abs," but this is a myth. The muscle that extends anteriorly from your rib cage to your pelvis is called the rectus abdominis. The separations you see across a defined six-pack are made by a fibrous structure called the linea alba. You cannot isolate a part of a muscle. You can, however, choose to do exercises that work the full range of the muscle belly and apply resistance to make the movements more difficult. Leg raises accomplish both.

CHANGE IT UP

Add a hip raise (by flexing your abs to lift your butt up at the peak of the movement) to turn this into a dynamic core exercise.

Hold a dumbbell between your feet or strap on some ankle weights as you get stronger.

> **Advanced:** Turn this into an expert-level isolation exercise by hanging from overhead bars rather than lying down. You'll have the perfect opportunity for this if you are training at a park!

Band Bicycle Crunches

Muscles internal and external obliques, transverse abdominals

This is a basic core exercise whose effectiveness can't be denied. Dropping down for a set of bicycle crunches is a great superset solution, and varying the tempo will keep your body guessing and adapting. It's manageable for beginners, but striving for perfect form creates a challenge for advanced exercisers.

INSTRUCTIONS

1. Wrap a band around your feet.

2. Lie back on a mat on the floor with your knees at a 90-degree angle, hands gently placed against the sides of your head.

3. Lift your shoulder blades off the ground by using your abs, being sure to keep a neutral spine. This is the starting position.

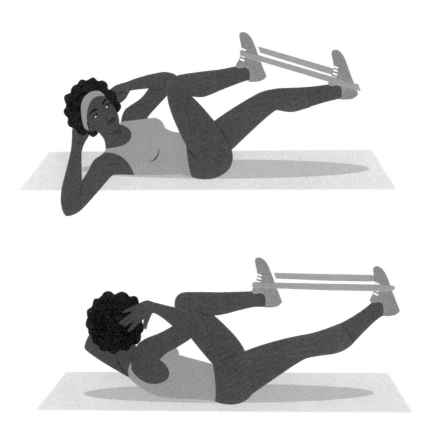

4. Engage your obliques to move your right shoulder up and press your right elbow into your left knee (left leg bends farther to get there). To balance, extend the right leg out at a 45-degree angle at the same time.

5. Reverse the movement to pass through your starting position and perform this action on the other side (left shoulder goes toward right knee). Your head will bob gently as your upper body shifts.

6. This is considered 1 rep.

COMMON MISTAKES AND HOW TO AVOID THEM

Avoid pulling on your neck. A good cue is to think about reaching for your knee with your shoulder and not your elbow. Remember, hands should lightly touch your head, not clasp it.

You will achieve a smaller waist if you work your transverse abdominals to compress your core during exercise. Though it is hard, putting extra effort into controlling your stomach during crunches will show in your results. This means engaging your abs by breathing out and pulling your belly button in before you start your set.

REMEMBER

Always do an equal number of crunches on each side.

CHANGE IT UP

To keep you from hitting a training plateau, make this exercise more challenging. You can do this by trying to pull your stomach further into your spine, switching up the speed of the sets, or by adding ankle weights.

> **Advanced:** This exercise works when done slowly, or as you get comfortable with form, when done more quickly! Blasting through a set of 60 bicycle crunches will boost your heart rate and help you burn away the fat that is keeping you from living your six-pack dreams.

V-Sit Twists

Muscles internal and external obliques, rectus abdominis, transverse abdominals, hip flexors

Performing this exercise requires core strength, balance, and coordination. Learning how to employ your abdominal muscles during twisting gestures is a practice that will safeguard your active lifestyle. Back strains often occur when people contort their bodies incorrectly, so practicing proper form is advantageous.

INSTRUCTIONS

1. Sit on a mat on the floor with your knees bent. Set your upper body in good posture—shoulders back, core engaged, chin up, chest open.

2. Clasp your hands together in front of you so your elbows are at 90 degrees, and press your upper arms against your sides.

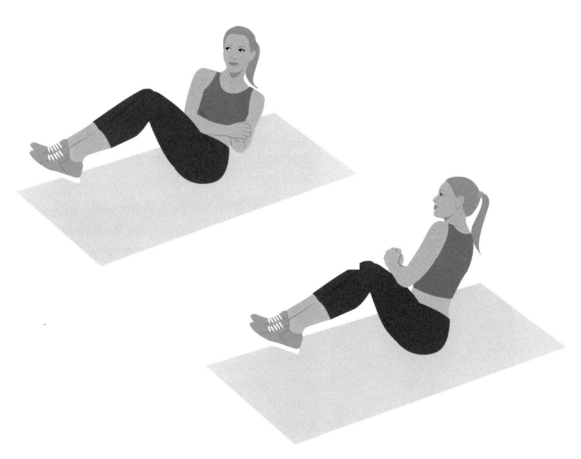

3. Shift your bodyweight back so your feet raise off the ground and you are balancing on your bottom. This is the starting position.

4. While maintaining equilibrium, twist your torso to the right by engaging your obliques.

5. Move back through the center to shift your upper body to the left.

6. This is 1 rep. Continue the specified number of reps, then rest after the set.

COMMON MISTAKES AND HOW TO AVOID THEM

Your upper body moves together as a locked group during this exercise, pivoting only at the torso, with your shoulders and arms held tightly at your sides. The head can either stay in place while you lock your eyes straight ahead (similar to "spotting" in dance terms) or you can inhibit neck function and let your face turn in the direction of your body.

Your lower back should be straight, which requires you to feel as if you are pushing it up and forward. Your form is off if your back is rounding and sinking back to the floor.

REMEMBER

A small range of motion is absolutely fine to start with. V-sit twists are a complicated action and require agility that takes time to develop. You should always do what you are capable of and be proud of yourself for progress. Eventually your midsection will be able to support your bodyweight to better hold the position and add movement.

CHANGE IT UP

The only way I would love this exercise more is if it was done on a downward angle! If you happen to do a workout at a gym with a decline bench, hop on and try doing oblique twists with gravity.

Advanced: Holding a medicine ball, dumbbell, plate, or other heavy object between both hands provides additional resistance.

Butterfly Crunches

Muscles rectus abdominis, transverse abdominals

Did you know that doing abdominal exercises improves digestion? This movement particularly burns calories and recruits your body altogether for better health. Opening up the lower-body limbs helps target your rectus abdominis for fuller range of motion and grounds you to the floor to reduce neck strain.

INSTRUCTIONS

1. Lie on your back and place the soles of your feet together, legs relaxed.

2. Maintaining control, lift your shoulders off the ground by contracting your abdominals, reaching your arms forward through your legs.

3. Squeeze momentarily and then relax back down to the floor.

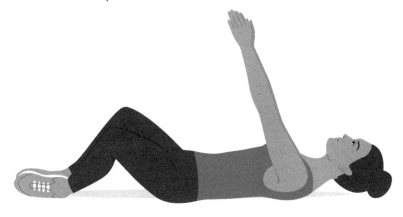

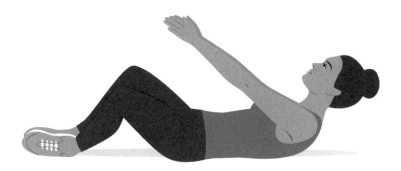

4. Repeat this action for the specified number of reps. Take 30 to 60 seconds to rest or perform a cobra stretch. (Lay on your stomach with your hands under your shoulders, then straighten your arms and lift your chest to stretch your abs). Then repeat for another 2 sets (or as specified in your fitness program).

5. Train your abdominals using isolation exercises such as butterfly crunches 2 to 4 times per week, with rest days to allow for muscle regeneration.

COMMON MISTAKES AND HOW TO AVOID THEM

- Never clasp your hands together behind your head; doing so can cause neck injury.

- The range of motion is not large—your goal is not to sit up completely but to raise your upper body partially off the ground.

REMEMBER

- The name refers to the placement of your legs—they fall open to resemble butterfly wings.

- This exercise is harder if you bend your knees more to bring your feet up closer to your buttocks. If you are having difficulty, try straightening your legs out slightly.

CHANGE IT UP

Intermediate: Pausing for a longer duration when contracted is beneficial for muscle endurance and strength.

Advanced: To move to a more advanced version of this exercise, lift your knees up as you crunch and reach your arms ahead through your open legs (above your feet). Fight to keep your knees apart and shoulders back to maintain good form.

COOL-DOWN EXERCISE
Planks with Shoulder Tap

Muscles transverse abdominals, rectus abdominis, internal and external obliques, deltoids, triceps, biceps, pectorals, trapezius, quadriceps, glutes, calves

This dynamic plank is a whole-body workout that builds exceptional core strength. It combines a fundamental isometric exercise with vigorous upper-body tasks to help you improve your muscle definition, balance, and coordination. It's a great finisher for both chest and core days.

INSTRUCTIONS

1. Kneel on a mat on all fours—knees under hips, hands under shoulders.

2. Start with your breath. Exhale deeply while focusing on drawing your abs in toward your spine to activate the transverse abdominals.

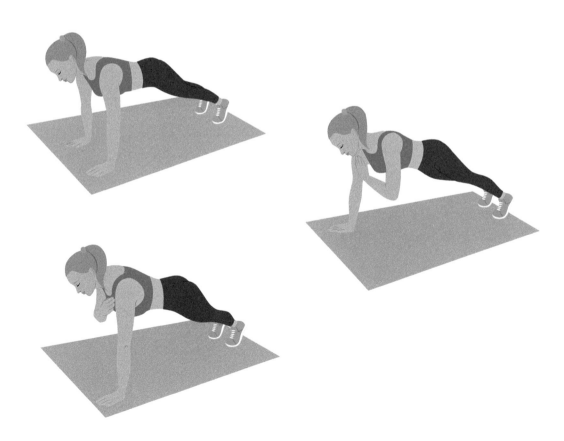

3. Continue to breathe while holding your tummy in. Slightly roll your shoulder blades back and squeeze them together.

4. Progress to a plank by extending your legs straight back and rising up on your toes. Don't drop down to your forearms but balance on your hands as you would for a push-up.

5. Plank with shoulder tap: Shift your weight onto your left arm and bend your right arm to tap your left shoulder using your right hand. Place your right arm back down and reach across your body using the left arm to tap your right shoulder.

6. Repeat this sequence for an equal number of reps per side.

COMMON MISTAKES AND HOW TO AVOID THEM

During a plank the lower back should not sag toward the ground, and the torso should not twist or bend. The goal with this exercise is to make the body as solid as a board while moving your arms.

REMEMBER

Speed is not encouraged here. You're going to struggle to hold this plank for the specified length of time, so rushing to tap faster is not advisable. Slow, controlled gestures will promote cell regeneration to help you achieve your fit physique.

CHANGE IT UP

Advanced: Place your feet on a BOSU ball or balance board to add another challenging component.

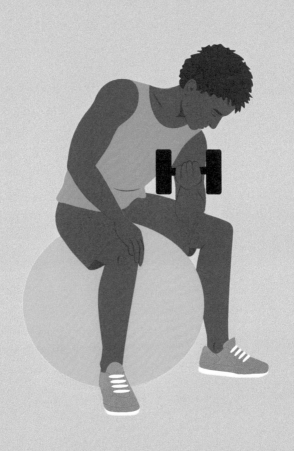

11

arms and shoulders

Defined, muscular shoulders and arms not only look impressive but they help you in other ways. Strong deltoids enhance your posture and give your body more stability. Strengthening your biceps and triceps will enable you to lift heavier weights during compound movements thanks to improved endurance.

warm-up exercise
Bent-Arm Lateral Raises

Muscles medial and anterior deltoids, trapezius

An athletic upper body is crowned by capped shoulders, and this is one of the primary exercises I credit for building up my deltoids. By bending your arms, you will be able to use heavier weights than with classic lateral raises, allowing for safe and effective overload of the movement.

INSTRUCTIONS

1. Stand facing a mirror and set up your body—chest open, shoulders pressed back, chin up, core engaged—while holding a dumbbell in each hand.

2. Bend your elbows to create a 90-degree angle while keeping your upper arms against your body and your forearms parallel with the floor. This is your starting position.

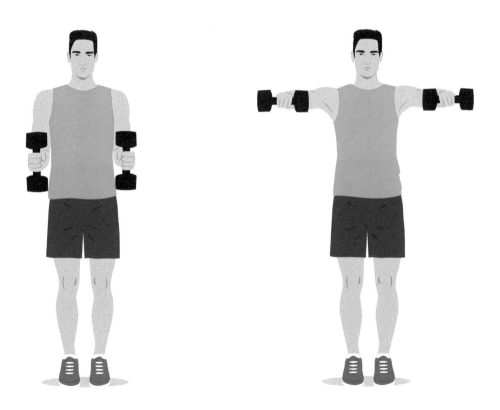

3. Lift your arms laterally away from your body. Raise them until your elbows are level with your shoulders.

4. Slowly lower your arms.

5. Repeat this motion immediately and continue it for the specified number of reps.

COMMON MISTAKES AND HOW TO AVOID THEM

When training clients, I often refer to this exercise as "tequila shots," because the raising of your arms with dumbbells mimics the action of a bartender holding two bottles to simultaneously pour shots. This will help you remember to keep your elbows locked at 90 degrees and not allow the dumbbells to come close to your chest—otherwise you will be dumping tequila all over yourself! Bad form in this movement looks like the chicken dance, so focus on your reflection in the mirror and watch to ensure your hands don't creep nearer to your armpits.

REMEMBER

Your best opportunity to improve strength is during the eccentric motion, or when you are lowering the weight with gravity. Focus on resisting the downward force to boost muscle development.

CHANGE IT UP

The shoulder complex intricately combines four joints and is the most mobile in the body, so it's absolutely imperative for you to spend time preparing it for activity. I pair light lateral raises with some reverse arm circles to create a well-rounded upper-body warm-up.

This exercise lends itself to being both a solid warm-up and a challenging working set. The best way to amplify this move is through drop-sets.

High-impact exercise
Shoulder Presses

Muscles medial deltoid, anterior deltoid, posterior deltoid, triceps, trapezius

The shoulder press is a fundamental bodybuilding lift that should be included in every good training program. It is one of the best ways to test your upper body strength and build power. Incorporating this movement in your training will also help pull back your shoulders to correct posture issues.

INSTRUCTIONS

1. Grab a set of dumbbells and take a seat.

2. Engage your core and roll your shoulders back to prepare for the lift.

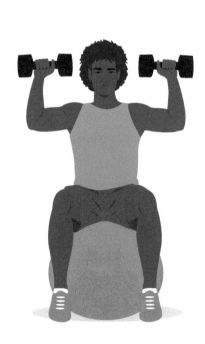 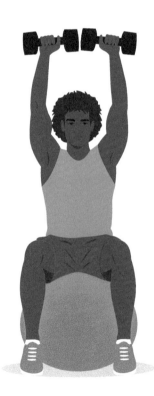

3. Bring the dumbbells together in front of your body and press them straight up overhead. Turn your palms to face forward. This is your starting position.

4. Bend your elbows so your arms lower toward your sides until they form a 90-degree angle.

5. Press the weight back up to the starting position. Perform the specified number of reps, or continue until your muscles fatigue and your form falters.

6. End the set with the dumbbells above your head, then turn your palms toward each other and slowly lower them in front, keeping your hands close to your body.

7. Rest for 30 to 60 seconds, then do additional sets as specified.

COMMON MISTAKES AND HOW TO AVOID THEM

- The setup for this exercise instructs you to begin and end the shoulder press in a way that safeguards your ligaments and tendons from tearing. Otherwise, the raising and lowering of the weights could place your shoulders in a position susceptible to injury.

- While keeping a neutral spine, you should be able to look up with your eyes and see the dumbbells when your arms are extended. If you cannot, correct your positioning and ensure that your press guides you along that new, slightly more forward pathway to protect your shoulders from repetitive use injury.

REMEMBER

- Doing warm-up sets and building up to your maximum lift is the best way to safely increase your muscle size and power. Never begin your workouts with your heaviest lift.

- Stretching lightly during rest periods makes the best use of your workout time and improves your mobility for better overall health.

CHANGE IT UP

Standing up incorporates more core stability to help you advance in your fitness.

> **Advanced:** Simply increasing the weight used is the best way to continue to see improvements in your physique.

Lying One-Arm Lateral Raises

Muscles rear and posterior deltoids

Sexy shoulders are complete only when nicely rounded at the back, which is accomplished through posterior deltoid isolation exercises like this one. Exercising your shoulders using a variety of movements is the only way to evenly build strength and muscularity. By lying down, you remove the temptation to swing your body to assist in the lift.

INSTRUCTIONS

1. Lie on your side on a bench or mat, and support your neck with your bent arm.

2. Choose a lightweight dumbbell and hold it using the arm closest to the ceiling.

3. Extend your arm out straight in front of your face, palm downward. Keep your shoulder pressed back.

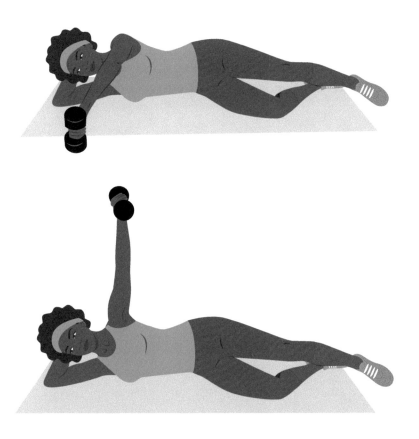

4. Squeeze your posterior deltoid to raise your arm perpendicular to the floor. Your working arm remains straight during this movement.

5. Lower the arm back to the first position and repeat the movement for the specified number of reps.

6. Rest, then switch sides to complete 1 set.

7. Continue to alternate sides to complete equal reps and sets per side.

COMMON MISTAKES AND HOW TO AVOID THEM

It's easy to allow tension to build up in your neck as you strain to do this movement. You can avoid injury by lifting a reasonable weight and focusing on the isolation of the posterior delt as the priority. Getting caught up in how strong you are for exercises like this is silly and unnecessary. Save your 1-rep maximums for compound movements like the shoulder press.

REMEMBER

- Training at home is super convenient, but you need to focus on safety. Whenever you're performing exercises in a lying position, even simple ones like this lateral raise, have your cell phone nearby in case an unexpected injury occurs. Having help within arm's reach should be a comfort.

- It's not necessary to lower the weight past parallel. Range of motion for this exercise is from eye level in front of your body to the arm straight up in the air. Your shoulder shouldn't be stretched at either end of this motion.

CHANGE IT UP

This movement could feel awkward at first. Instead of holding your working arm out straight, you could try bending your arm to form a 90-degree angle, your wrist even with your elbow, and performing the one-arm lateral raise while maintaining this position. Locking your arm with the elbow bent makes the exercise easier by shortening the lever.

Bicep Curls, Standing Partial

Muscles biceps

Another name for this true torture is "21s." This challenging biceps exercise will take your arm definition to a new level, and it's tough to cheat. The instructions will help you coach yourself through muscle fatigue and push your body to break through training plateaus for amazing results.

INSTRUCTIONS

1. Stand with shoulders back, core tight, holding two dumbbells at your sides. Palms can either be supine (facing up) or in hammer position (neutral position, with palms facing your body). I personally find that hammer position is more comfortable and protects my wrists from unnecessary strain.

2. Bend your arms to bring the dumbbells all the way up to your shoulders without moving your upper arm.

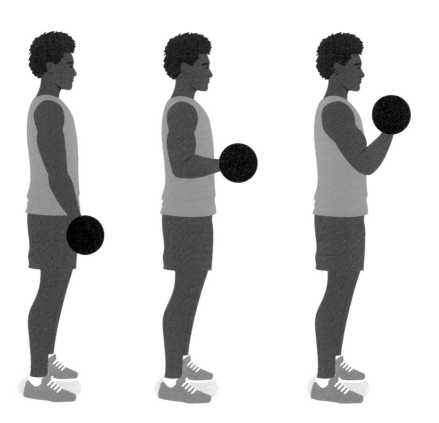

3. Lower the weights back to your sides, but don't allow your arms to rest.

4. Lift the dumbbells again for 7 full reps.

5. Immediately raise the dumbbells up to begin the next group of repetitions. This time, lower the weight only to elbow height, forming a 90-degree angle with your arms.

6. Perform 7 half reps through this upper range of motion.

7. On your seventh half rep, allow your arms to extend down to your sides, but still don't allow your biceps to slack.

8. Start the next partial repetition and lift the weight halfway up, creating a 90-degree angle with your arms.

9. Lower the weight to your sides and do 7 final reps in this way.

10. Finally, you may relax your arms and put down the dumbbells for about a minute before starting the next set of 21s.

COMMON MISTAKES AND HOW TO AVOID THEM

Your arm above your elbow does not move at all during this exercise. Having your upper arms glued to your sides prevents you from swinging the dumbbells to use momentum to accomplish the lift.

REMEMBER

You can actually do this exercise in any order. I find the lower half of the partial reps to be the most difficult, and personally prefer to leave that for the last 7 reps, but you can get that out of the way first, and all the reps will be just as effective.

CHANGE IT UP

Advanced: Stand with your back against a wall to force yourself into a good posture and to take away the opportunity for you to sway your body during this action.

Overhead Tricep Extensions

Muscles triceps

To increase the thickness and shape of your arms and impact all-around strength, leave time in your upper body workout to isolate your triceps. Strong triceps create stability in your shoulders and arms, which greatly improves your ability in compound lifts such as the shoulder press.

INSTRUCTIONS

1. Stand, or sit, on a stability ball or bench with one dumbbell held in both hands.

2. Raise the weight overhead, palms facing up. You should be holding one end of the dumbbell rather than gripping the handle, to keep your wrists in a neutral position. Your upper arms should be held against the sides of your head.

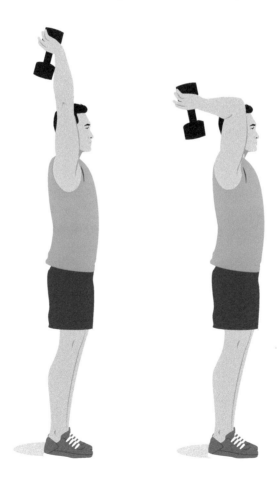

3. Allow the weight to descend behind your head. Your forearms should be about parallel with the floor.

4. Squeeze your triceps to lift the dumbbell back toward the ceiling.

5. Repeat the number of reps specified in your fitness program before resting.

COMMON MISTAKES AND HOW TO AVOID THEM

Be cautious you don't overextend the shoulder joint during the decline phase of this exercise. You should not feel a pull or pain, but if you do, stop immediately and consult a doctor before resuming the movement. Engage your core before lifting the weight and continue to hold the contraction to protect your spine until the dumbbell is safely returned to the floor during your rest period.

REMEMBER

Single-arm overhead tricep extensions are more challenging, so reduce the weight if you decide to isolate one side at a time. It's a good idea to stabilize your body by crossing your free hand in front of your body and holding your working upper arm in place during the sets.

CHANGE IT UP

You can easily perform this exercise using bands if you are training with limited equipment. Loop the band around the fingers of one hand, and lock that arm up behind your head. Lift your other arm—this is your working arm—up against your head and bend at the elbow to hold the other end of the band. Open up the elbow so your working arm points straight up. Slowly lower only the forearm in the reverse motion to return back to the previous position. This action is explained in free exercise tutorial videos on juliegermaine.com/90-day-plan.

Concentration Curls

Muscles biceps

Flexing your biceps shows off your great arms, so targeting this group of muscles is an obvious must. Your biceps will grow as a result of back training, but you will be happier with the outcome of your fitness program if you also spot-train your arms regularly.

INSTRUCTIONS

1. Sit on a bench, stability ball, or chair with your legs open. Hold one dumbbell in your right hand. Visit juliegermaine.com/90-day-plan to see how to set up this exercise with a glute band.

2. Bend forward at your hips, ensuring your back is completely straight.

3. Lean your right arm against the inside of your right thigh to secure your body. Hold your left thigh with your free arm to further stabilize yourself.

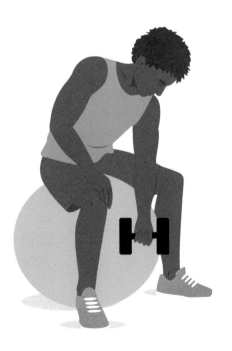 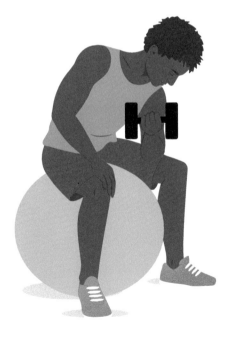

4. Curl your right arm to bring the dumbbell to your chest.

5. Squeeze your biceps for extra intensity, then slowly lower your arm to hang open again. The magic of this exercise lies in the eccentric motion. Take your time and control the tempo to your benefit.

6. Repeat additional reps to fatigue the muscle and immediately reverse your posture to train your left arm.

COMMON MISTAKES AND HOW TO AVOID THEM
This exercise enables you to control the alignment of the movement, so you can shift your weight back as your body adapts to put more stress on the biceps, creating a setup similar to that of a preacher curl.

REMEMBER
This is a movement that's safe to take to full muscle failure, so push yourself! Your set should be complete when you literally cannot lift the dumbbell again and have to drop it to the floor. You also have the option to crush your arms with drop-sets.

CHANGE IT UP
Use a glute band for concentration curls by looping one end around the foot opposite to your working arm.

> **Advanced:** You can change up which head of the biceps takes on more load during each rep by rotating your wrist between the supine and hammer positions (see instructions for bicep curls, standing partial on page 158).

Arnold Presses

Muscles deltoids, biceps, triceps

Since this variation of the basic overhead press requires rotation, it works many different muscles in the shoulder joint and arms. The twist of the palms to face backward from the forward position while lowering the dumbbells targets the anterior deltoids and increases the range of motion, which steps up muscle growth.

INSTRUCTIONS

1. Sit on a stable bench, preferably with a back support. Hold two dumbbells in your lap. (You can also use a stability ball, but be even more diligent to contract your core—your strength will be inhibited, and the weight used should be decreased.)

2. Take a breath and set your shoulders back, chest open. Maintain a neutral spine and engage your core.

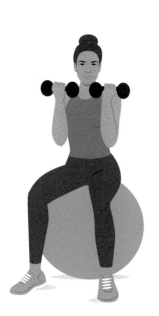
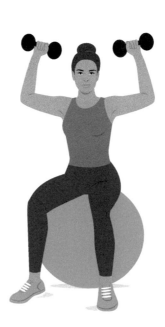
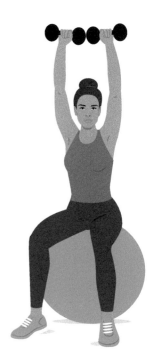

3. Lift the dumbbells up to your chin, palms facing your chest and held close to your body. (Later you will return to this posture to complete each rep.)

4. Exhale as you press the dumbbells upward, gradually turning your hands so the palms face forward by the time they pass eye level. Your elbows open up your arms to the sides.

5. Continue the movement fluently to fully extend your arms overhead in a shoulder press.

6. Inhale and reverse your moves back to step 3.

7. Complete the specified number of reps. Between sets, lower the dumbbells to the floor and lightly stretch your shoulders and torso.

COMMON MISTAKES AND HOW TO AVOID THEM

You move through the standard overhead press position when performing the Arnold press. Your elbows should go from straight down under your wrists at the start to out by your sides to create a 90-degree angle in your arms halfway through, and your arms end up straight above your head.

REMEMBER

If you suffer from shoulder injuries or feel shaky at all during this exercise, avoid doing it and revert back to a more comfortable and safe movement.

CHANGE IT UP

You can perform standing Arnold presses by stabilizing yourself with your feet shoulder-width apart and activating your glutes. Having a strong core is essential.

Advanced: Make this exercise harder by starting with your upper arms parallel to the floor, dumbbells at eye level. In this case, you move your elbows laterally to open up the chest while rotating your wrists to face palms forward. This alternation keeps pressure on the front of the shoulder consistently during the entire exercise.

COOL-DOWN EXERCISE
Plank Walks

Muscles anterior and medial deltoids, triceps, pectoralis major, trapezius

The plank is such a fantastic exercise for muscle development, core strength, and physical endurance that I've provided a few variations. Plank walks give a great challenge to the upper body while keeping your workout really fun and dynamic.

INSTRUCTIONS

1. Place one band around your upper arms and another around your thighs, just above the knee.

2. Drop to the floor and take a plank position (see page 148), balancing on your hands.

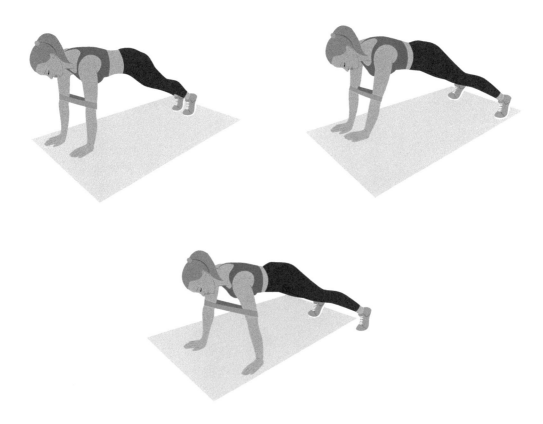

3. To move to the right, step your right foot out and follow by lifting your right arm to move your body a step in that direction.

4. Walk your left leg in to touch your right leg, then lift your left arm to move it next to your right arm.

5. Continue to travel sideways in this manner across the floor as far as you can in the available space.

6. Walk laterally in this manner in the other direction.

7. If your room is small, you may be able to go back and forth only a few paces.

8. Time yourself or perform equal repetitions on both sides.

9. Rest, then repeat.

COMMON MISTAKES AND HOW TO AVOID THEM

- Balance is a factor during this exercise, so it's acceptable to start with tiny increments and work up to larger movements to maneuver back and forth.

- Try to keep your hips level with the floor and your body stable. Rocking around clumsily shows a lack of core strength and will improve with practice.

- Don't hold your breath!

REMEMBER

Though you want to look to make sure you are not going to bump into anything, do try to keep your chin tucked down and your spine in a neutral position.

CHANGE IT UP

Advanced: Wall walks are a challenge waiting for you! If you're bored of planks and feel like blasting your delts in a new way, give this a go. Do a plank on your hands with your feet near the wall. By stepping with both your hands and feet, move your body up the wall until you are in a handstand position, or as near to one as you feel comfortable attempting. Hold, then walk yourself back to the ground. This advanced exercise can be made more difficult by doing a push-up at the start and a handstand push-up at the end.

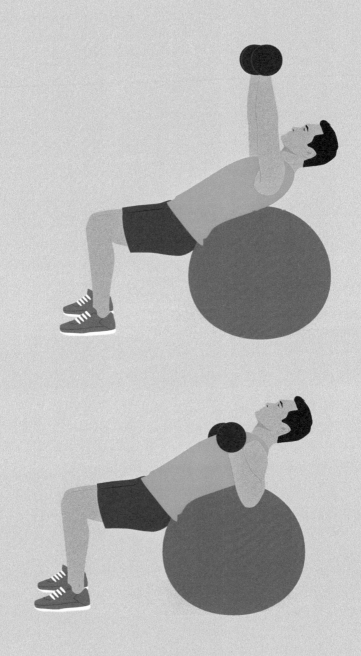

12

chest

Both men and women profit from incorporating chest days into their weekly training schedule. Improving your posture with strong pectorals helps your breathing and lifts breast tissue by building the muscles beneath the tissue. Your job and daily activities are made easier when you have strong chest muscles, because the chest is involved with many different movements, like pushing, lifting, carrying, and holding.

warm-up exercise
Push-Ups

Muscles pectorals, triceps, abdominals, anterior deltoids

Love it or hate it, this simple exercise is extremely effective at improving the muscularity through your chest, shoulders, and arms. It is also so easy to incorporate and can be a great warm-up for any workout. Drop and give me 10!

INSTRUCTIONS

1. Get into the starting position by facing downward on the floor, your weight divided between the balls of your feet and your hands. Your back stays straight throughout the movement and your head faces down.

2. Bend your elbows and lower your body, creating a 90-degree angle with your arms. You may need to adjust your hand position if they're not underneath your elbows.

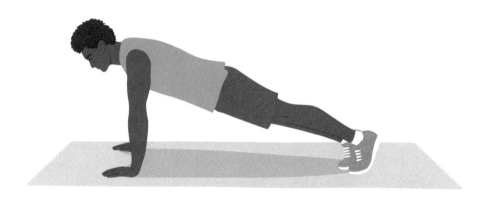

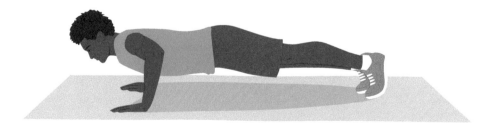

3. Squeeze your chest and press back up to the starting position.

4. Repeat until failure or as specified in your fitness program. If you are a beginner, you can bend at your knees to reduce the bodyweight.

COMMON MISTAKES AND HOW TO AVOID THEM

- Your head shouldn't hang toward the floor but should be facing down and held in a neutral position to protect your spine.

- It's common to allow the lower back to sink as you fatigue. Fight this bad habit by contracting your core and not releasing it until you reach the rest period.

REMEMBER

- Don't shrug your shoulders or let gravity quickly pull you down.

- Your hands should be on a firm surface to protect the wrists and safeguard you from slipping. If you want to have a more neutral position, you can purchase push-up bars. Push-up bars keep you from putting additional strain on your forearms and the tendons in your wrists.

CHANGE IT UP

Intermediate: Drop-sets of push-ups to fail are a fantastic way to encourage muscle development. Keep in mind that when you reduce the bodyweight by bending at your knees, your form through your core and upper body should hold.

Advanced: Ask your workout partner to load a plate onto your back to add resistance to the push-up when calisthenics aren't enough for you anymore. You can also use a dumbbell on top of a towel across your upper back and have your buddy hold it in position—or a small child can hop on for a fun ride!

High-Impact Exercise
Chest Presses

Muscles pectorals, triceps, abdominals, anterior deltoids

Building up to an impressive bench press is a goal for many men and women. To accomplish this, you must incorporate the chest press in your training at least once a week and ensure your form is correct to bolster strength gains and muscle regeneration. Results will come quickly if you are dedicated.

INSTRUCTIONS

1. Grab two dumbbells and take a seat on your stability ball.

2. Step your feet forward and allow the ball to roll up your back so your chest faces upward. Keep the dumbbells held tightly together in front of your body as you get into position.

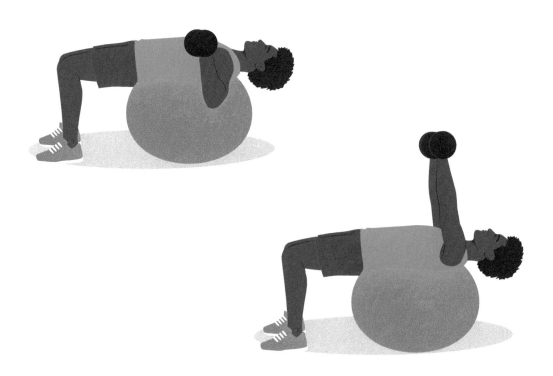

3. Press the dumbbells straight up together and set yourself up with your wrists and weights aligned. This is your starting position.

4. Bend your elbows to a 90–degree position, lowering them sideways, breathing in as you do so.

5. Using your chest, exhale and push the dumbbells up and together. You should feel a squeeze in the middle of your chest at the very top of the movement.

6. Complete reps to muscle fatigue (not failure) and rest before repeating for the specified number of sets.

COMMON MISTAKES AND HOW TO AVOID THEM

- The bench press, or chest press, is a compound movement that gives you a fantastic core workout. Engage your abdominal muscles before starting your set for best results.

- Warming up before this exercise is very important, and you can do this with lighter sets that lead to your heavier ones. Never start with your working set, as you can cause muscle tears that will take months to recover from.

REMEMBER

You will be focused on increasing the weight used while maintaining proper form and can expect to graduate from doing this exercise on a stability ball to needing a supportive flat bench. In a pinch, an aerobic step with risers can be used as a bench.

CHANGE IT UP

Try one arm at a time to test your core strength and gauge any muscular imbalances. Lock your free arm into place by putting your hand on your thigh. Your shoulders should be set back and pressed down during the exercise, even on the side that is not loaded.

When training in a gym, you might want to do bench presses under a barbell. Always use a spotter for safety and start with the bar at eye level, then lift and press over your nipples.

Chest Flys

Muscles pectorals, anterior deltoids, abdominals

Opening up your chest using flys is a great way to improve your posture and range of motion for a variety of exercises. Having tight pectoral muscles leads to upper- and lower-back pain, causes neck issues, and limits your strength gains due to bad lifting form.

INSTRUCTIONS

1. You will need two dumbbells and a stability ball.

2. Get into position by engaging your core and setting your shoulders back and down, neck aligned with a neutral spine.

3. Roll down the ball to support your back and press the dumbbells overhead with your palms facing each other.

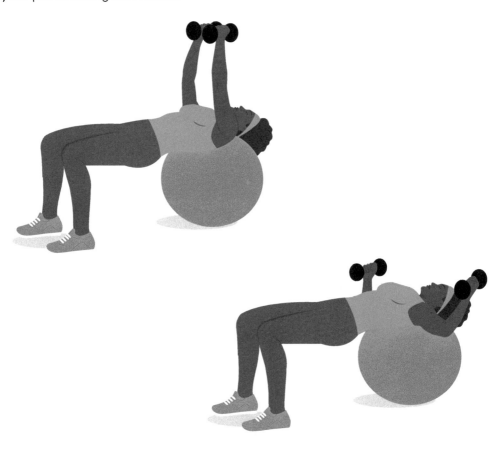

4. Bend your elbows slightly.

5. Lower the weight laterally—but not below your body—until you feel a pull in the chest. Your arms don't bend farther and should remain slightly bended.

6. Squeeze your chest to return the weights overhead.

7. Repeat until you reach the repetitions specified in your workout. Rest and repeat for the desired number of sets.

COMMON MISTAKES AND HOW TO AVOID THEM

- Don't lock the elbows. The straighter your elbows are during the movement, the more strain and stretch are applied to the pectoral muscles. So during your setup, note the slight bend recommended in the arm and hold your body in that position for the entire set.

- It's always a good reminder to breathe during your set, and a good workout partner will cue you to do so—exhale when raising the weight, and inhale when lowering.

REMEMBER

- If you suffer from tight pecs, don't try to overextend your chest using heavy weights. You will benefit from checking your ego at the door and choosing a reasonable dumbbell, or even no weight, to start off with while your body adjusts to the new movement and eases into a fuller range of motion.

CHANGE IT UP

You can bend your hips to drop your lower body farther toward the ground with your back on the stability ball to create an inclined chest fly position. This targets the anterior delts and makes your body work in a new way, which encourages strength and size gains.

Incline Chest Presses

Muscles pectorals, anterior deltoids, triceps, abdominals

The purpose of this exercise is to target your anterior deltoids and develop your upper pecs for more muscle fullness and size. Changing the angle of the standard chest press works your body in a way that promotes cell regeneration and adaptation, which leads to a stronger, better physique.

INSTRUCTIONS

1. Hold two dumbbells while you are seated on a stability ball.

2. Activate your core and roll your shoulders back, pressing them down firmly.

3. Roll yourself to a lying position, bending your hips to form an incline rather than a flat angle with your body.

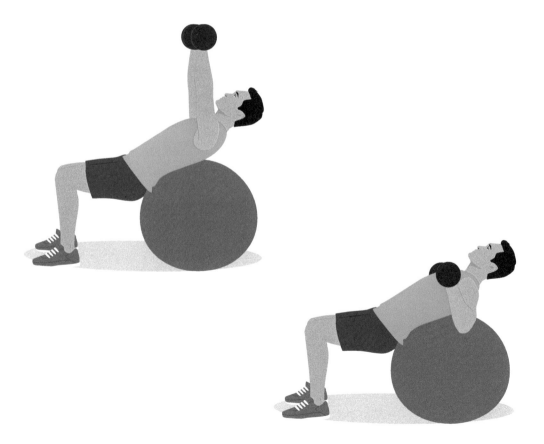

4. Push the weights up to the starting position, arms straight above, palms facing forward.

5. Lower the dumbbells until your arms create a 90-degree angle out to your sides. Don't overextend the shoulder joints by going lower than 90 degrees.

6. Using your upper-body strength, exhale as you push to extend your arms above you.

7. Repeat and rest as specified in your exercise routine.

COMMON MISTAKES AND HOW TO AVOID THEM

- Due to the pressure of your back pressed into the ball, you may want to set yourself up near a wall so the ball doesn't fly out from under you. This means sitting down rather than rolling to prepare for the exercise, so be cautious of how you turn to pick up the weights. Awkward reaches can lead to back injury and muscle strains.

- Cocking your wrists backward when holding weights is not good practice. In other words, forming a 90-degree angle at your forearm and hand puts a lot of pressure on your tendons and will lead to an overuse injury with time. Don't forget neutral body positioning in any area, including your hands.

REMEMBER

- To target the upper chest without the shoulders dominating, the best angle from flat is 30 degrees.

- Use your shoulder blades to anchor your upper body and help you attain the right form to get the most out of this exercise. It helps to think about leading the movement from your elbows, pushing from under rather than over.

CHANGE IT UP

If you don't feel comfortable in the inclined position on the stability ball, replace this exercise by re-creating the same angle with decline push-ups, in which you elevate your feet on a ball, couch, or chair.

Tricep Push-Ups

Muscles pectorals, triceps, anterior deltoids, abdominals

This variation is significantly tougher than standard push-ups and puts prominence exactly where you would assume: on the triceps! Also known as close-grip push-ups, this exercise works wonders for building endurance, strength, and size in the upper body and trunk and requires no equipment at all.

INSTRUCTIONS

1. Position your hands side by side on the floor, about 3 inches apart. Extend your legs so you are balanced face down on your toes and straight arms. Be sure to engage your core by breathing out and pulling your stomach in and up. Your neck will resist gravity to maintain a neutral spine, and your shoulders should be pressed back and down. The knees are locked to keep the legs straight.

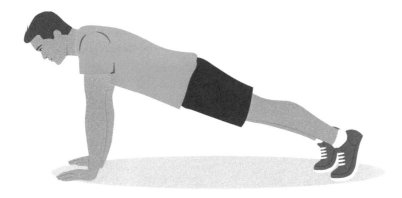

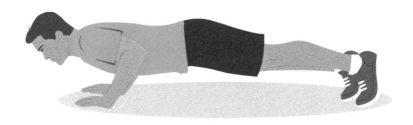

2. Bend your elbows while holding the rest of your body perfectly still. As you lower yourself slowly toward the floor, inhale. The arms remain much nearer to the body than they would in a typical push-up.

3. Exhale and exert force through your hands to elevate your body back to the starting position.

COMMON MISTAKES AND HOW TO AVOID THEM

- Some coaches will instruct you to position your hands together on the floor barely touching to form a diamond with the pointer fingers and thumbs underneath you. Don't do this. Your hands need to be only slightly closer than shoulder-width apart.

- Full range of motion recruits the muscles in the chest and arms for optimal progress. If you aren't able to drop your chest close to the ground, consider doing tricep push-ups from your knees to start with and moving to your toes once your strength allows you to.

REMEMBER

The imbalance from bringing your hands closer than shoulder-width apart for this movement is what makes it special. You are still going to be a step closer to your goal if you gradually inch your hands together over the weeks, so don't be discouraged if this exercise is too advanced for you.

The rigid plank form necessary for any good push-up translates well into many other exercises and benefits your overall fitness. Take time to learn how to isolate and engage the muscles in your core and keep those techniques at the top of your mind.

CHANGE IT UP

Elevate your legs on a ball or bench to distribute more weight to your upper body when calisthenics become too easy for you.

COOL-DOWN EXERCISE
Chair Dips

Muscles triceps, anterior deltoids, pectorals

If you want stronger arms, bench (or chair) dips are the solution. This versatile exercise can be done anywhere and is adjustable for every fitness level, providing a great muscle building effect. Attention to proper body positioning truly makes all the difference in your fitness results, and dips will help you develop good alignment.

INSTRUCTIONS

1. Sit down on a stable chair with your hands resting on the front edges beside your thighs.

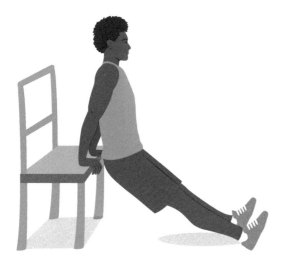

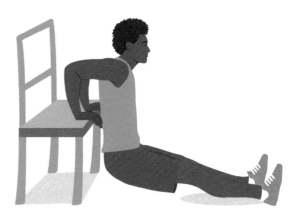

2. Move your feet forward so your butt lifts off the chair and hangs out in front. The ideal starting position for chair dips is with your legs straight out in front of you, but it may take time to achieve this, so a bend in the knee is also completely okay.

3. Hinge at your elbows to form a 90-degree angle with your arms, resulting in your body dropping down in front of the chair. If your butt hits the seat, shift yourself forward to allow clearance.

4. Push through your palms to lift your body back up to the straight-arm starting position.

5. Immediately begin another rep to complete the set as specified in your fitness program, then rest and repeat for the desired number of sets.

COMMON MISTAKES AND HOW TO AVOID THEM

- During this action, your arms should graze by your body rather than flaring out to your sides. This helps not only to better target the triceps but also to protect the shoulders from trauma.

- Speed is bad here, so take your time and make your muscles work to control the ascent and descent of your body.

- If you feel pain in your shoulders, consider how low you are going and correct bad form by allowing your upper arms to be parallel to the floor, no closer.

REMEMBER

- This exercise is great as a superset or part of a fitness circuit. In these cases, you would not rest after the set but would follow the guideline regarding what exercise to do next.

- If you have a shoulder injury or limited range of motion in that joint, you should choose another exercise until you are fully recovered and have your doctor's approval to return to chair dips.

CHANGE IT UP

By bending your knees, you take burden off your upper body and place it on your lower body, allowing you to do the movement with less effort. Work up to performing dips with straight legs, and then challenge yourself with additional resistance by placing a weight securely on your upper thighs.

wrapping it up

Congratulations! You have completed an intense 12 weeks of training and should be very proud of yourself. It takes a dedicated person to stick to a workout program and follow a restrictive diet for any length of time.

To achieve big goals, you must focus all your attention and spend large amounts of your time working on them. Fitness aspirations, in particular, can put a strain on your body and life beyond what is sustainable long term. For this reason, it's important to put the brakes on and give yourself some space to fully recover and find balance again.

A period of rest is part of your program now that the main portion of the plan has ended. Your body will benefit by taking a full one to two weeks off from physical activity, after which you should replace aggressive training with light workouts. Return to exercise by incorporating low-volume movements at high repetitions and gradually resume your normal fitness routine.

The reason for this pause is to give both your mind and muscles time to recuperate from the high level of performance you demanded. Athletes can experience overtraining injuries or burnout if this aspect is overlooked.

You can make the most of this downtime by giving your body all it needs to promote muscle recovery. Continuing to eat high-protein meals and drinking plenty of water is a good start. Don't overdo it by indulging in high-calorie, high-fat foods. Instead, revert back to a diet similar to that of Week 1, with regular cheat meals. Adequate amounts of sleep are key—aim for seven to eight hours a night. Stretching is advantageous and is one of the best things you can do to prevent future injuries. Now may be the ideal time to increase your dexterity by working on your mobility every day for 10 to 15 minutes. Spending time foam rolling tight problem areas or indulging in a deep tissue massage is also a great way to work out knots in your muscles and ease soreness in your joints.

Yes, it's true that it can be extremely hard to slow down and shift your mindset, but recovering 100 percent from your program will be worth the effort.

weigh-in chart

Name   **Date**
_____

Measurements

Weight (lbs)   Height
_____

Skinfolds Measurements (mm)

Triceps   Chest
_____

Midaxillary   Subscapular
_____

Suprailiac   Abdominal
_____

Thigh
_____

Bodyfat (Methods)

Jackson / Pollock
_____

Continued on next page

Continued from previous page

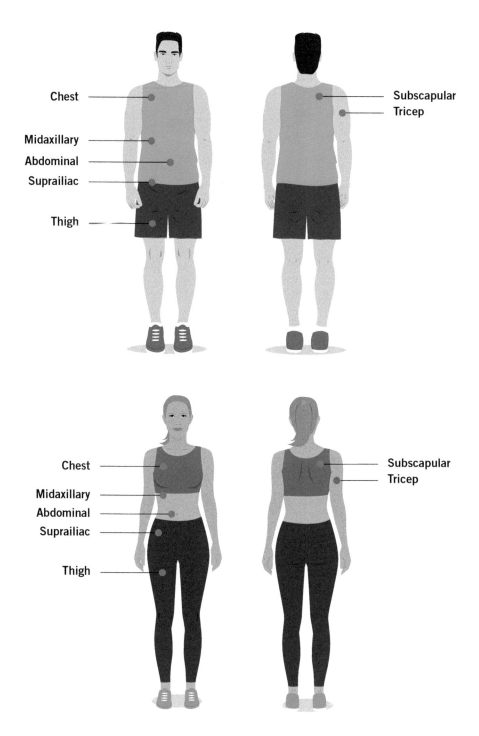

Chest

Midaxillary

Abdominal

Suprailiac

Thigh

Subscapular
Tricep

Chest

Midaxillary

Abdominal

Suprailiac

Thigh

Subscapular
Tricep

Resources

Julie Germaine Coram Fitness Online Resources:

- Calorie Calculator: juliegermaine.com/90-day-plan
- Exercise video tutorials and other useful information to support you in your fitness transformation: juliegermaine.com/90-day-plan
  - › Improving flexibility/stretching: juliegermaine.com/stretching-how-to-get-flexible-fast
  - › Motivation, healthy recipes, and more: juliegermaine.com/fitness-blog
  - › Online fitness program sign-up: sweatwithjulie.com
  - › Setting up a great home gym: juliegermaine.com/great-home-gym
  - › Strength charts: juliegermaine.com/charting-your-strength
- Product store to order all the equipment needed: juliegermaine.com

Other Useful Resources:

- American Council on Fitness. *ACE Insights Blog.* acefitness.org/education-and-resources/professional/expert-articles.
- Contreras, Bret, and Glen Cordoza. *Glute Lab: The Art and Science of Strength and Physique Training.* Canada: Victory Belt Publishing, 2019.
- Delavier, Frédéric. *Strength Training Anatomy*, 2nd ed. Champaign, IL: Human Kinetics, 2005.
- Schwarzenegger, Arnold, and Bill Dobbins. *The New Encyclopedia of Modern Bodybuilding.* New York: Simon & Schuster Paperbacks, 1999.

Index

Acknowledgments

I am truly grateful for the opportunity to help so many people through this platform. Thank you to the entire team at Callisto Media, particularly my editor, Andrea Leptinsky, for making my goal of becoming a successful published author achievable, and for guiding me and giving me such a wonderful project to focus on during a terrible pandemic. Much love and appreciation to my parents for their endless support, especially my beautiful mother and proofreader, Rose-Marie Coram. Finally, though she is just a toddler, thank you to my daughter, Amelia Rose Coram. I will cherish the memory of writing this book while watching you dream, during these happiest of days together.

About the Author

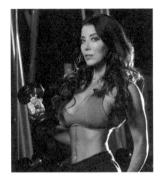

Coach **Julie Germaine Coram** has devoted her life to her passion for fitness and to helping others reach their goals. She is an expert on fitness competition preparation, but her true mission is to guide everyday people to find happiness in balanced, active lifestyles. Julie is a full-time mother, cookbook author, and entrepreneur who celebrates her good health daily by bike riding, weight training, and inline skating with her young daughter. It is important to Julie to be a good role model for her family, friends, and millions of online subscribers. This international fitness champion is also certified in prenatal and postpartum fitness and absolutely loves coaching new and expecting mothers to introduce baby to the world in the best possible way. Via her website juliegermaine. com, Julie offers one-on-one online fitness consulting to clients around the globe, and since 2005 has helped myriads of men and women successfully reach their goals and enjoy better health.